A foreign correspondent in medicine

Rob Stepney

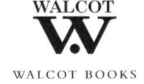

WALCOT BOOKS

ISBN 978-0-9538442-2-7

Charlbury 2020
Copyright Rob Stepney

Published by
Walcot Books
2 Walcot Farm Cottages
Charlbury OX7 3HJ
01608 810180

www.robstepney.com   robstepney@outlook.com

Book designed in Charlbury by Keith Rigley
Printed by Henry Ling Ltd, Dorchester

Acknowledgements

I am grateful to Geoff Watts and David Loshak of *World Medicine*, Tim Radford and John Illman of *The Guardian*, Celia Hall of *The Independent*, and Corinne Short of *Medical Monitor* – all of whom published early articles. Karol Sikora and Howard Smedley helped me understand cancer, and we wrote a book together. In cardiology, similar thanks are due to John Wallwork, with whom I wrote another book. John Thompson and Heather Ashton taught me enough pharmacology to understand the basics of how drugs work. Christina Surawy kept me up to date with cognitive therapy. I am also grateful for her love and support over the years, and to Nick, Eva and Trystan, who helped with this book, and to whom it is dedicated.

As explained in the introduction, the idea stems directly from Kieran Cooke's *A Not So Foreign Correspondent in Ireland*. I happily acknowledge that debt, and I greatly appreciated his experienced encouragement when writing a couple of pieces for Radio 4's *From Our Own Correspondent*. This book was designed by Keith Rigley in Charlbury, which is an extraordinarily creative place in which to live.

Contents

	Introduction	7
One	**Immortality, but at a price**	9
	Immaculate dissection	9
	What does Henrietta Lack?	13
	Immortal, divisible	17
Two	**Teaching intimate anatomy**	22
	Vaginal examination – the professional approach	22
	Consent now central to intimate examination	26
Three	**HIV and herpes: viruses we've learned to live with**	30
	Boxing HIV into a corner	30
	Turning HIV against itself	32
	Herpes spread reaching epidemic proportions	37
Four	**Affairs of the heart**	42
	Four hours to beat the clot	43
	Hope springs eternal: the coronary stent	46
	The dawn of statins	49
	Turning back the clock	50
	Engine and gearbox: another Cambridge first?	51
	For the man having a heart attack on platform 1	55
	Snake venom is an ACE solution	57

Five	Murder most foul, or murder most foolish?	62
Six	Beauty and the bombs	70
Seven	Being male means being mortal	75
	Spotlight on men's health	75
	Let's just measure your aorta, sir	80
Eight	Matters in mind	83
	An Icelandic saga	83
	Writers of insight and insanity	84
	I'm not Diogenes, I just collect things	89
	How one man panicked, and survived	93
	Accentuate the positive	96
	Eliminate the negative	98
Nine	Not all brilliant ideas have a bright future	101
	Finding the way home	101
	Is there anything there?	103
	String theory	109
	Backing up the heart	112
	Spurt in artificial blood	115
	Parkinsonism's great leap forward	118
	Bone marrow banking "could soothe nuclear fears"	121
Ten	Cancer: playing the long game	124
	Cloning a killer for the front line	128
	Sense of tumour failure	132
	Counting on the cancer clock	135
Eleven	Danger: doctors at work	139

Contents

Twelve	**A fertile furrow**	144
	A series of unfortunate events? Mortality in a Borsetshire village	144
	Sex, scandal crime ... Ambridge is just following national trends	150
	Doctor with his finger on Ambridge's pulse	151
Thirteen	**A long view of the gut**	155
	Poetry in motion	155
	Can you catch an ulcer?	156
Fourteen	**From Virginia to vaping**	160
	Homo fumens	162
	Cigars and Sigmund	164
	It's not a patch on sucking	169
	Smoke signals	172
Fifteen	**QALYs become the metric of medicine**	176
Sixteen	**Communication key to better care**	180
	Videophone offers long-distance diagnosis	180
	Breaking down the barriers	182
Seventeen	**Taking drugs and alcohol on board**	185
	The real inside story	185
	Drunk? But not a drop passed my lips	189
Eighteen	**Speculations in obstetrics**	193
	The ultimate test tube baby	193
	Can a foetus feel pain?	198

Nineteen	**Christmas crackers**	203
	Ding dong merrily on high, fly by with Santa's mushrooms	203
	Healer, dealer, heart stealer: portrayals of the doctor in popular music	207
	Back to the future: how good are doctors at gazing in the crystal ball?	212

Index	221
Books by Rob Stepney	228
About the author	228

Introduction

In November 2014 I was reporting from a meeting abroad when an e-mail arrived from a friend back home in Charlbury: Did I know that I was being credited with having "invented" the word vaping? And then came a mail from a friend in Ann Arbor, Michigan, asking the same question.

When Oxford Dictionaries made "vaping" their word of the year, the earliest example they could find of its use in print was in a *New Society* article I had written in 1983. As it happened, I'd also used the term in a *Guardian* piece in the same year.

I don't know whether I really did coin the word – quite an obvious one in the circumstances – or whether I heard someone else use it. Far more important than the word was the idea of the device itself (which I had no part in formulating); and the fact that – even though a very good idea – it was such a long time in coming to fruition.

That is the way of many things in medicine, and science generally. It has been a privilege to see on many occasions the painstaking process by which good ideas eventually bear fruit, but it has been sobering also to see its opposite – when ideas that seemed good at the time turned out not to be so. I think of artificial blood, of adding muscle (literally) to the heart, and of chronotherapy in cancer. Their time has still not come, and it may never arrive.

Some things in medicine are like that. Other ideas bear fruit amazingly quickly. Examples would be antiretroviral drugs to combat HIV, thrombolysis to dissolve clots during a heart attack, and coronary stents.

A *foreign correspondent in medicine*

I have had the good fortune to spend forty years as something like a foreign correspondent in the land of medicine: able to flit about what was most interesting at the time, irrespective of the specialist area. And so there is something on cancer and on cardiology, on an infamous case of a surgeon who murdered his wife, on HIV and herpes, on being a Northern Ireland GP in the time of troubles, on a digital alternative to dissection and other kinds of immortality. On all of it, I have been able to take a long-term view, but I have not revised in hindsight what I wrote at the time.

I would not have had the idea for this book without Kieran Cooke's excellent *A not so foreign correspondent in Ireland* (Killsalagh Press 2018). This is a series of reminiscences from a man who, though born Irish, is sent to Ireland as a foreign correspondent for the British press. This alerted me to the idea that being a foreign correspondent is not always an uncomplicated concept. In my case, I want the book's title to convey the idea that, although I've spent most of my professional life in and around medicine, I have never been fully part of it, having always had at least one foot in another camp.

This was perhaps most evident early in my work as a journalist. Richard Wakeford, a friend from the Clinical School at Addenbrooke's Hospital in Cambridge, alerted me to the fact that medical students were being taught vaginal examination on anaesthetised women who had not consented. Chapter 2 picks up the story.

Chapter One

Immortality, but at a price

It became clear that there were several unintended ironies in this first piece. Death from drug overdose was not what I was imagining at the time I wrote it; nor was the "perfect man" at all perfect. The fact that I describe a source as being "coy" about the details suggests I had an inkling of an unusual, perhaps even macabre, twist to the tale.

IMMACULATE DISSECTION

The Independent on Sunday September 1993

Accurate anatomy is the father and mother of medicine, but can it be learned without a scalpel? In Denver, Colorado, the corpse of a "perfect man" is being stored on computer disc.

Earlier this month, a committee of American doctors convened by teleconference to arrange a kind of immortality for a very special corpse. Its anatomy will be electronically archived for posterity with a thoroughness and detail never before attempted. Every facet of the face, each nook and cranny of the body, every bit of bone, every twist and turn of intestine will be preserved. True, only as digital information: but who is to say that God has any more reliable form of data storage?

A *foreign correspondent in medicine*

For most of us, the end of our material remains will come either quickly among flames or as slow underground decay. For the chosen male cadaver now in a cold store at the University of Colorado Health Sciences Center in Denver, physical destruction will be by a milling machine which grinds it away millimetre by millimetre from head to toe. But before each cross-sectional slice of tissue is removed, its appearance will be preserved on video and photographic film and the images stored on disc.

For Dr Victor Spitzer, a specialist in medical imaging, and for anatomist colleague Dr David Whitlock, this month's decision brings them to the end of a two-year search for a perfect specimen of man. "The committee considered two males that suited our purpose. They were both great, with no disfiguring trauma or surgery and no diseases that altered the anatomy," says Dr Spitzer. It took the panel just thirty minutes to decide which of the two candidate cadavers would be chosen for the "Visible Human Project". The vacancy for an ideal female is still open.

Literally, the candidates must be in good physical shape: average weight for height, aged between twenty and sixty, race immaterial. They must also have willed their bodies to science. The lives of people considered must have ended in a non-destructive way. So what *did* the ideal corpse die of?

Dr Spitzer is coy about the details. But, early on it became clear that some form of non-violent suicide would be appropriate. "After drug overdose, people are not suitable donors for organ transplantation and are therefore good candidates for us. But the need for autopsy means we lose some," he says.

"There has been a lot of grey humour needed to keep us sane," admits Dr Michael Ackerman, who oversees the

Immaculate dissection

million-dollar Visible Human Project for the US National Library of Medicine. He recalls that when universities were asked to bid for the job of finding suitable bodies, the phrase "putting out a contract" was used with care.

"More than ninety percent of bodies willed to science end up in the dissecting room," says Dr Spitzer. "This is really just an updating of a time-honoured concern with anatomy as a tool for medical teaching and research."

Before subjection to the milling machine, cross-sections of Denver man will be recorded by magnetic resonance imaging (MRI), which records the structure of fat and muscle particularly well. The anatomy will then be imaged slice by electronic slice using X-ray computed tomography (CT). Photography comes at a late stage when the body is cooled to minus seventy degrees centigrade and pictures are taken as each millimetre-thick section is ground away. The whole painstaking process will take about four months.

The CT and MRI images will be stored along with digitised versions of the photographs, and all can be called up together and compared. The computer will be able to "stack" adjacent sections allowing 3D images to be constructed and explored. Anyone wanting to study the heart, for example, can call it up on screen, either whole or section by section.

The intention is that the imagery will be publicly available both on the planned "data super highways" spanning the nation and on compact disc (CD-ROM). But the undertaking is vast. Only one CD is needed to store the 59 million words in the twenty volumes of the *Oxford English Dictionary*. But the Visible Human will require seventy.

A dissecting room without bodies may seem paradoxical, but medical students of the future could study anatomy by dismembering an electronic corpse rather than the real thing. All will be there except the feel of the scalpel and the smell of formalin.

Donors' real names will not become known. But, perhaps predictably, they have already been dubbed Adam and Eve. "Adam and Eve were not necessarily typical humans but they were the first of the line," says Dr Ackerman. If the first digitised humans prove as useful as he thinks, they could soon be joined by a whole family of digitised people, from conception to old age.

Postscript

Despite the assurance of anonymity, it soon became clear that the male cadaver used in the project was that of Joseph Paul Jernigan, a 39 year-old executed in Texas on August 5th 1993 by lethal injection. Jernigan admitted to having knifed and shot a man whose home he had robbed. The story is that a prison chaplain persuaded Jernigan to donate his body to science, but there was probably no explicit consent to its use in the way outlined above. The *Visible Man* dataset was released in 1994 and the *Visible Woman* a year later. Both have been widely used: licences for access were granted to four thousand people or institutions from sixty-six countries. From 2019, access no longer requires a licence.

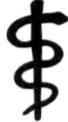

WHAT DOES HENRIETTA LACK?

World Medicine September 1982

A woman who died decades ago lives on throughout the world.

In February 1951, a biopsy was taken from the cervix of a 31-year-old woman from Baltimore who had complained of spots of blood appearing between her periods. Although the 2.5cm soft purple lesion had not looked like cancer, it was found to be malignant. Within eight months, the woman was dead.

It is known that her first name began with the letters HE, and her surname with LA. It is also widely agreed that she was black. But much else has been in doubt. What is not disputed is that the cells from HeLa's biopsy have now [in 1982] been alive for over thirty years since their donor died.

In this time, they have adapted so well to laboratory cultivation that HeLa cells seem surreptitiously to have taken over almost every other cell line available. HeLa had the opportunity to contaminate everything in sight because it was so widely used: for the culture of viruses (such as polio, which requires primate cells in which to multiply), and as a research tool in protein synthesis and genetics.

The sheer volume of her cells must now be so great that a small village could be populated entirely with HeLas. Even ten years ago, the *Medical Journal of Australia* calculated that their weight would exceed that of their donor. Another estimate was that HeLa would have taken over the world if allowed to grow unchecked under optimal conditions.

A missing reference?

The "birth" of HeLa was the work of George Otto Gey, a distinguished cell biologist who worked at Johns Hopkins University. In their initial 1952 report, Gey and colleagues described how a human cancer had been grown for almost a year in a medium of chicken plasma, bovine embryo extract and human placental cord serum. That success – the establishment of the first human cell line – followed years of failure. The report is still given as the source reference for HeLa cells, despite the fact that it is only an abstract of a conference paper. Its few sentences give no details of the donor, nor of what made her cells so special.

There is evidence that Gey did write a more complete account, but, oddly it seems never to have been published. A 1953 paper cited it as "in press" with the journal *Cancer Research*, but the paper did not appear in any volume of the journal published over the next five years. And no reference is made to it again.

Helen Lane by any other name

The question of HeLa's identity was raised in 1973 by John Douglas, of Brunel University, who wrote to *Nature*. On the occasion of HeLa's "coming of age", he suggested, it was time her true name was revealed.

His letter prompted a reply from Howard W Jones Jr, who drew Douglas' attention to a 1971 paper he had written in the journal *Obstetrics and Gynecology*. In this article, Jones tells the story of HeLa's first visit to the Johns Hopkins outpatient gynaecology department and reveals that her name was Henrietta Lacks.

What does Henrietta lack?

Douglas accepted that the question of HeLa's identity had been resolved. She was not after all Helen Lane, as many had supposed, nor Hedy Lamarr, nor Helga Larson, nor Heather Langtree, as had also been suggested. The *Medical Journal of Australia* also seemed satisfied that "the lady who has achieved test-tube immortality" was Henrietta Lacks.

But Helen Lane did not go away so easily. A year later, the *Medical Journal of Australia* was back with a leading article in which the cells' donor was once again named Helen Lane. And most people who work with HeLa cells seem to have clung to the original identification.

There *are* some slightly odd things about Jones' claim that HeLa was Henrietta. First, he does not mention that the donor was black. This, along with the fact that HeLa was female, had always been generally accepted. Secondly, Jones and colleagues claim that the original diagnosis of her tumour was wrong: the cancer was not epidermoid but an aggressive adenocarcinoma. Had the diagnosis always been wrong, or had Jones et al been looking at a different kind of tissue?

Then there was a strange experience which raised the possibility that the new name was a macabre joke. I was talking about the renaming of Helen Lane to Charles Barnes, who is involved in tissue culture at the Cambridge University Department of Obstetrics and Gynaecology. "Henrietta Lacks," he said. "Isn't that part of a children's skipping song? I think it goes:

Henrietta Lacks
Henrietta Lacks
What does Henrietta Lack?
A body."

Of men and monkeys

Contamination of cell cultures is not rare. There are instances where cells purportedly from human tissues turn out to be those of monkeys, rats and hamsters. But HeLa's extraordinary ability to contaminate other lines is particularly embarrassing. Biologists who think they have been working on tissue from an entirely different source suddenly find that at some point it had been taken over by HeLa. Years of work can be lost.

The latest edition of the *American Type Culture Collection Catalogue* lists 85 cell lines which were ostensibly derived from non-HeLa sources but which turn out to have characteristics unique to HeLa cells. Dame Honor Fell, a pioneer of organ culture and a friend of George Gey, has said, "The HeLa cell has only to look at another culture to colonise it."

Others cite sloppy laboratory practice. David Franks, of the Cambridge Pathology Department, blames mistakes and mislabeling, and bottle caps which unscrew when placed in liquid nitrogen, allowing cells to escape. Once contamination has occurred, it is difficult to trace back. Scientists carry cell lines round in their brief cases to swap at conferences, or send them through the post. The paths by which cell lines are acquired are as complicated as race horse pedigrees, but largely unrecorded. Dr Franks commented: "Even originators have lost their own line and got it back from someone else."

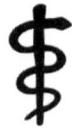

Twenty years later, the ownership of cell lines had become an important question and Henrietta Lacks was still centre stage.

IMMORTAL, DIVISIBLE
The Independent March 1994

Henrietta Lacks died 40 years ago but her cells live on and multiply. They are a marvel of microbiology but also an ethical and legal minefield.

Little is known about Henrietta Lacks except that she lived in Baltimore, Maryland, and died of cervical cancer at the age of 31. Long after her death, she has become the unsung heroine of modern cell biology by achieving a curious form of immortality. Although Henrietta died in 1951, her cells live on in thousands of test tubes in hundreds of laboratories around the world.

Months before her death, doctors took a sample of tissue from Henrietta's cervix, and George Otto Gey, from Johns Hopkins University, managed for the first time to grow human cells continuously outside the body. In culture, they would survive and divide, potentially forever. Henrietta Lacks' cells are called the "HeLa" cell line. Since they derive from a common ancestor, their genetic uniformity provides scientists with an element of predictability in research.

There are now many thousands of lines derived from different people, and they have proved invaluable in the study of disease. Cell lines are also crucial to the development of an increasing number of pharmaceutical products, and this has raised the question about who owns them. Are the original cells the property of the donor? Or the scientist or company who immortalised them? Or nobody?

The European Collection of Cell Lines, housed near Salisbury, Wiltshire, contains more than ten thousand, each obtained from individual patients or healthy volunteers. A principal function of the collection is to keep the frozen cells free from contamination.

An early problem with the HeLa line is that it was so good at growing in nutrient broths, it ended up growing where it wasn't supposed to – often as a result of scientists failing to sterilize their equipment. Many lines, such as HeLa, derive from tumours. The abnormal ability of these cancer cells to divide in the body means they have a natural tendency to grow in lab culture. Another and recent way of creating a line is to infect a human cell with a virus or fragment of viral DNA – a process called immortalisation.

Human cells in culture have potential in the manufacture of new and expensive medicines, like interferon, derived from our own immune system. Ray Spier, professor of microbiology at Surrey University, says these complex proteins can be obtained by other means such as inserting human genes in rodent cells or bacteria. "But the drugs will be more faithful copies of substances found in our own bodies if they are made using human cells," he explains.

The Wellcome Foundation uses the Namalwa cell line, originally obtained from an African child with a form of lymph cell cancer prevalent on that continent, to produce interferon. The child could have had no conception that millions of her cells would be used to manufacture a potentially life-saving drug on an industrial scale.

Human cell lines also have advantages in the production

of vaccines. Two lines in particular, both obtained by immortalising human lung cells, are used to manufacture vaccines against rabies, measles, mumps, German measles and hepatitis A. "We used to be scared by the theoretical possibility of inducing cancers by using cells that grow continuously in culture," Ray Spier recalls. "But extensive testing has failed to show any significant risk."

Human cell lines have produced great benefits for all, and, for some, considerable profits. Now, the ability to immortalise cells is adding a difficult twist to the already tangled debate about the ownership of human tissue and the limits of its legitimate use.

When John Moore developed a rare form of leukaemia, he was admitted to the University of California Medical Center in Los Angeles under the care of Dr David Golde. To slow progress of the disease, Moore agreed that his enlarged spleen should be removed. With a potentially fatal disease, he may have thought it unimportant, but on the consent form for surgery he declined to allow the university the right to exploit cells from his tissues.

Nevertheless, John Moore's spleen cells were cultured so that they would grow indefinitely. Four years later, California University set out to patent the immortal cell line. Dr Golde and the university subsequently sold exclusive rights to exploit the line to the Genetics Institute Inc and the drug company Sandoz. The package of cash, fees, and shares Golde and colleagues negotiated was reportedly worth $3 million.

Moore's cells were thought to be a valuable source of lymphokines, natural substances that control aspects of the immune system. It was recognised that immortalising the cells had added value to them. But was the process akin to making wine from grapes, in which case Mr Moore had merely provided the raw material? Or could he make a more substantial claim, based on the fact that the cells were still in essence his property – like other parts of his body?

By a majority decision, and to the surprise of those involved, the California Supreme Court ruled that a patient retains no property rights over body tissue removed during surgery and later used to develop new treatments. But the court did accept there had been impropriety in exploiting Mr Moore's cells against his express wish and gave him the right to sue for failure to obtain consent and breach of trust. Moore eventually settled the case for what was described as a relatively modest sum.

In the UK, the rights of the patient from whom cell lines derive have never been tested. Does that person have a legitimate interest in any profits made by a doctor or drug company? Money aside, can patients retain any say over how their living cells are used?

Diana Brahms, a barrister specializing in medico-legal matters, has some sympathy with the potential claim of patients. "When you allow tissue to be removed, you probably take the view that it will eventually be incinerated," she says. "You would rightly be upset if the tissue was used for a purpose you disapproved of. If research were done without your consent and to the financial advantage of the doctor, it would be neither lawful nor ethical."

Molecular biology is advancing at such a pace that the potential use of human cell lines can only be guessed at. Cloning a human from the unique genetic makeup in each of our cells is a highly remote prospect. But it was with this in mind that a scientist discussing Henrietta Lacks once suggested, only half in jest, that she should have put $10 in an investment account in 1951, and waited.

Postscript

Rebecca Skloot's 2010 book *The Immortal Life of Henrietta Lacks* became a best seller, won many prizes for science writing, and was the basis of a film. Henrietta's daughter Deborah is reported to have said that her mother's hand guided its writing.

On the wider question of ethical and legal responsibilities for the creation and use of cell lines, the Human Tissue Act of 2004 introduced a complex system requiring consent and licensing, but the exact provisions vary depending on the nature of use and whether or not the source of the material is anonymised.

Medical Research Council guidance emphasises several relevant principles. Researchers should ensure that the wishes and interests of the donor are respected. The human body and its parts shall not give rise to direct financial gain. Intellectual property rights arising from research using human biological samples may be sold or licensed. But it is not appropriate for a company to be given exclusive rights to a collection of samples made with the benefit of public funds.

Chapter Two

Teaching intimate anatomy

In 1983, Richard Wakeford, a friend from the Clinical School in Cambridge, alerted me to the fact that medical students were being taught vaginal examination on anaesthetised women who had not consented. Both Richard and I thought this a scandal, and I questioned the practice in an article for the weekly magazine *World Medicine*. I confess that I did not confront the practice as forcefully as I should have done in that first piece: medics I knew, and even my girlfriend who was then a junior doctor, could not understand why I was making any fuss at all. How else should students learn?

I was rather more robust when I returned to the topic ten years later. Happily, by that time, much had changed.

Vaginal examination – the professional approach

World Medicine November 1983

However much doctors view the vagina as just another orifice, for the lay person it is an emotionally charged piece of anatomy. Concern is growing about whether medical students should be learning how to examine it by using an anaesthetised patient who has not been asked to consent. Using a paid "professional patient" is now the American way. Would its adoption be helpful here?

It is quite usual in Britain for medical students to make their first fumbling attempts at vaginal examination on an unconscious patient, and the General Medical Council report on basic medical education shows that students on gynaecology attachments find theatre sessions valuable for this reason. The vicious cycle of mutual embarrassment is avoided. An initially heavy hand causes no discomfort. And there is good opportunity for a more experienced colleague to instruct on technique.

Disquiet about whether it is ethical to teach on a woman without her explicit consent is stilled by the vital need for students to be taught, and the fact that patients in the future will benefit from their learning. Besides, in a teaching hospital, the patient will already have consented, or at least not objected, to being examined by medical students in other contexts. Even if the patient might feel unhappily vulnerable about being examined while unconscious, she does not know about it. So where, doctors ask, is the problem?

The difficulty is that patients *are* likely to see something of an ethical dilemma. This is partly because of the particular significance attributed to their reproductive organs, but mostly because they are in hospital to be treated, and this practice would seem like using them as a teaching aid.

For all that doctors might disagree, Ian Kennedy, professor of medical law and ethics at King's College, London, sees it that way too.

"On one hand you've got the desire and need to train people, and on the other you've got a clear invasion of the privacy and integrity of the woman. And the latter should be paramount," he says. "Admittedly, it can be said it doesn't harm her. And on one level it doesn't. But what if she finds out and feels she's been, figuratively, raped?

"The doctor in charge might well be judged to have acted unethically. He or she may also have acted illegally because this would be an assault. If the patient was not told, she can't have consented."

Professor Kennedy is not impressed by the idea that in accepting treatment at a teaching hospital patients are implicitly agreeing to students taking part in their treatment: "I've never been persuaded of that argument," he says. "I don't think you give blanket consent like that. You don't generally choose the hospital, you go where you're sent And you certainly don't abandon all rights to privacy when you get there."

But one senior registrar, with responsibility for teaching, says: "Professor Kennedy offers a counsel of perfection in legalistic terms. If we took everything he said seriously, we'd get nothing done."

Perhaps because the American consumer movement is more vocal, American doctors have had to cope with these problems for some time. Justifying a new approach, Robert Kretzschmar five years ago wrote in the *American Journal of Obstetrics and Gynecology* that the patient was "exploited by the teaching system as student examinations at this level do not contribute to patient care".

One American innovation is the professional patient — an informed, experienced and relaxed mannequin ready to tell students if they are feeling what they are supposed to feel, whether or not it hurts and, above all, whether their manner is going to put patients at ease. Another is the recruitment of

Vaginal examination – the professional approach

"gynecology teaching associates," who are mostly health professionals or graduates in behavioural science, and are either completely healthy – so that the range of normal variation can be experienced – or women with stable though abnormal features.

All are trained in vaginal examination or anatomy. Pay in 1979 was around $12 an hour, judged an educational bargain because of the saving in physicians' time. Use of such surrogate patients has spread to over fifty medical schools and independent assessment of students taught by them shows an advantage over traditional methods.

Might the idea be useful to us? A gynaecologist at the Elizabeth Garrett Anderson Hospital says she finds the money idea "slightly repulsive". She also doubts the teaching value of a few sessions with a trained patient. Dr Gerald Swyer, chairman of Women's Health Concern, is also sceptical about the idea of paying people. "It raises a big question mark about the nature of the women prepared to sell themselves for teaching purposes."

Ian Kennedy sees some virtue in the American way: "The US makes commerce out of most things. It would probably be exploitation of women who need the money – but that's a different question."

Jean Robinson, a lay member of the General Medical Council, is also in favour. "A large number of women don't like vaginal examinations," she says. "But the medical profession has taken extraordinarily little interest in finding out what it is that women most dislike and how things might be improved.

"The American system of having an awake, aware and consenting patient, who is actually teaching the doctor, is much better. You don't get feedback from an unconscious patient. Nor, of course, do you get consent. "

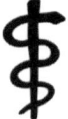

CONSENT NOW CENTRAL TO INTIMATE EXAMINATION

The Independent April 1994

Teaching students to examine the vagina using unconscious women who have not given their consent has been the tradition in Britain. It is a practice that is ethically unacceptable, legally questionable and of uncertain educational value.

Thankfully, the traditional approach is changing. But it was not until last year [1993] that the British Medical Association issued guidelines making clear that anaesthetised women must not be used as unconsenting teaching tools. The BMA's handbook *Medical Ethics Today* now contains the explicit statement that teaching hospitals should obtain prior written consent for vaginal examination of anaesthetised patients.

Gynaecologists at Dudley Road Hospital in Birmingham were among the first to introduce express consent. The move followed research which showed, without exception, that women objected to not being asked.

"We now make clear that only one medical student will perform the examination and we require that the student introduces him or herself to the patient beforehand," says David Luesley, senior lecturer in obstetrics and gynaecology at Birmingham University. Following this frank approach, only 10–15 per cent of women refuse permission.

Learning vaginal examination is a vital part of training. It is a skill necessary in taking a cervical smear, in investigating most gynaecological complaints, in many family planning procedures, and in the care of women in pregnancy and labour. A decade ago, when the issue of consent to examination under anaesthetic was first raised, gynaecologists argued that their ability to teach would be jeopardised by any change in practice. This has not happened.

"If anything, the system now makes teaching easier, since everyone feels more comfortable," Mr Luesley comments. "We have proved we can adopt explicit consent without compromising training."

This view is confirmed by Richard Beard, professor of obstetrics and gynaecology at St Mary's Hospital Medical School in London. In the St Mary's department the standard consent form for anaesthesia now asks women if they will give permission for up to two medical students to examine them in the operating theatre. "In six years, only three women have refused," Professor Beard says. "It is important to show respect for patients, and this has not interfered with the need to teach."

Change has also been welcomed at Addenbrooke's Hospital in Cambridge. "In some teaching hospitals, it used to be that as many as half a dozen medical students would line up to examine a woman under anaesthesia," says Steve Smith, professor of obstetrics and gynaecology. "Now a student in our hospital is allowed to examine a woman under anaesthesia only if he or she has personally asked the patient's permission beforehand.

"The change is a good example of the need for the public to raise issues which some gynaecologists had not even thought of, and for the profession to be responsive."

Jean Robinson, a lay member of the General Medical Council for 14 years, has closely followed the issue of consent to gynaecological examination. She believes the growing number of women in medicine has also played a vital part in changing attitudes.

"Obstetrics and gynaecology is still male-dominated, and that is not the way the public would wish it," she says. "But the teaching of vaginal examination has benefited from women medical students raising the issue. Now that women form half the medical school population, you no longer have to become a pseudo man to survive."

Nevertheless, Mrs Robinson is still concerned about the "quality" of consent obtained from patients. "Many women feel they are not in a position to refuse," she argues.

It may be that American experience has something to offer here. Richard Wakeford, a specialist in medical education from Cambridge University, collaborated in a survey of students from the United States and Britain to find out how they had gained their first experience in vaginal examination. Forty-six per cent of the UK sample said it had been on an unconscious patient. In America, the figure was 2 per cent. More than two-thirds of the US sample had first been taught the skill with the co-operation of a volunteer who was not a patient. In the US, hired subjects now teach examination of the male genitalia and rectum as well as examination of the vagina.

David Luesley agrees that it is valuable to have someone who can explain in clear terms what is comfortable and what is not. But he has his doubts about adopting the American system. One concern involves finance. "In the United States, teaching associates are paid, and it is not clear where the resources would come from in this country," he says.

His other concern is the artificiality of the situation. "Though well-trained instructors would be able to give good feedback on what hurts, they would probably not show the same anxiety and embarrassment as a typical patient. Overcoming this, as much as learning the anatomy, is crucial to the skill of vaginal examination."

Chapter Three

HIV and herpes: viruses we've learned to live with

When you've seen one pandemic, you've seen one pandemic. That is an epidemiologist suggesting that we can't learn much about how to deal with Covid-19 from pandemics of the past, even respiratory ones. But is it true? Looking back to the time of the HIV/AIDS pandemic, which was different in nature but also involved a retrovirus, gives some grounds for hope and some for pessimism: on the one hand, we developed effective treatments in a very short space of time; on the other, we still have no vaccine – and that is not for lack of trying.

BOXING HIV INTO A CORNER

Vancouver 1996, 11th international AIDS conference

"We have had episodes of hope before. Will this meeting really be seen as the turning point in the long struggle against HIV?" Waiting for a lecture to start, and needing to prepare a summary of the conference for the *AIDS Letter* of the Royal Society of Medicine, I had written that question at the top of my notepad.

"The answer to your question is 'Yes'," said the man sitting next to me. He was Julio Montaner, one of the conference's four co-chairmen. Later, I recounted that exchange in my report – and added "history will tell whether his optimism is justified". Happily, history has shown that it was.

Boxing HIV into a corner

San Francisco, some years earlier

This account relies on recollection rather than record, since my notes were never made public and I can no longer find them. But I recall being at a small meeting convened by a group of pharmaceutical companies which brought together medicinal chemists and virologists. Data were presented on the highly effective suppression of HIV replication using a number of different novel agents. But with each agent the virus quickly developed resistance, and blood levels of the pathogen bounced back.

For a while, I couldn't understand why the general mood in the room was optimism. Only gradually did I realise that those present had only ever been thinking in terms of using these new drugs as elements in *combination* therapy. That would be the future.

I remember one of the medicinal chemists asking the virologists to identify three points of vulnerability in the cycle of HIV replication. One weak point, as we knew, would not be enough. And the virus was also likely to mutate itself around two mechanisms of inhibition. But having drugs that acted at three different points in its cycle would very likely put HIV in a box from which it could not escape.

Not long later, after the chemists had designed molecules to target the three weaknesses the virologists had picked out, we had "highly active anti-retroviral therapy" or HAART – which slashed the death rate from AIDS and turned HIV into an entirely manageable, albeit still incurable, disease.

We now have several classes of anti-HIV drug which have different mechanisms of action and can be used in various combinations. The early agents, like AZT, stopped viral RNA being translated into the DNA which was then incorporated into the DNA of our own cells. These were the nucleoside reverse-transcriptase inhibitors. This class was joined by inhibitors of the various viral enzymes needed to assemble new viral particles.

Pharmaceutical companies have at times been accused – with reason – of disease-mongering: of over-inflating a problem for which they have a solution. To a man with a hammer, everything looks like a nail. But that San Francisco meeting was the situation in reverse. There was a problem in desperate need of a solution. And, within a remarkably short space of time, the companies delivered.

Of course, they were motivated at least in part by the demand for profit. But that imperative works. And it is one that could usefully be deployed against Covid-19, or multiply drug-resistant bacteria, for example.

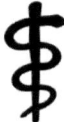

In 1995, I wrote a piece on progress against HIV. Some of it turned out to be close to the mark.

Turning HIV against itself

The Guardian May 1995

Can drug combinations cause the virus to mutate into a manageable infection?

It is paradoxical, but the unrivalled ability of the HIV virus to become resistant to drugs may be its undoing. False dawns have been so frequent in AIDS research that people have stopped looking at the sky for signs of hope. So far, the Human Immunodeficiency Virus has been able to counter anything we have thrown at it. But there is now the prospect that we can make HIV infection a manageable disease.

Let us start with the problem. Far from lying dormant for many years – as was once thought – it is clear that HIV reproduces itself at an incredibly fast rate. In an infected person, there are half a billion new viruses produced each day. And each time a single virus particle replicates, it introduces a change in one of the 10,000 elements that make up its genetic code.

This means that every possible mutation is generated thousands of times daily. It is therefore small wonder that HIV evolves ways of resisting drugs.

Those viruses that mutate in a way which makes them drug resistant survive. But the changes that they introduce to escape treatment make them at least marginally less well able to reproduce. Otherwise, evolution would already have selected for those mutations.

So, by using different combinations of drugs to manipulate the mutations HIV comes up with, it should be possible to convert it into a form that is weak enough to be kept permanently under control.

It is now clear that the changes that confer resistance to one drug sometimes inhibit the development of mutations to another. This is seen when the new drug 3TC is given together with the old drug zivodudine, or AZT. The initial impact on HIV is profound, the number of viral particles in the blood dropping by 99%. More importantly, the ability of the virus to recover from this dual attack seems severely curtailed. Levels in blood remain around 90 per cent less than before, and stay that way for at least a year.

This is almost certainly because the mutation HIV uses to escape the effects of 3TC makes it more susceptible to AZT. But is even 90 per cent suppression of the virus sufficient to allow the infected person to survive?

This year has brought the first clear evidence that the immune system is in fact surprisingly good at combating HIV. The virus is indeed replicating at an enormous rate, but the immune system is eliminating the virus almost as fast. It is only slowly that HIV gains the upper hand.

If we can shift the balance in favour of the body by repressing virus production, it should be enough to reverse the outcome of the struggle. "Immune reconstitution may be possible as long as replication of the virus can be held in check," says Dr Simon Wain-Hobson, of the Institute Pasteur in Paris.

The key will be to treat the disease early on, using several different drugs at once. "By early, I mean within the first few months of infection. We don't yet have the drugs which are safe and effective enough to do this, but it is foreseeable within five years", says Dr Jan Albert of the Swedish Institute for Infectious Diseases Control.

The evidence from these virus resistance studies is one reason for the optimism of scientists involved in HIV research. Another is our increased understanding of what happens in those rare cases of people who are repeatedly exposed to HIV but whose bodies successfully clear the virus. There are now many well-documented cases of such people. They include not just Kenyan and Gambian prostitutes but also babies born to HIV-positive mothers and health care workers accidentally injected with infected blood.

In some people, exposure was to weakened strains of the virus. But others survive because of a strong immune response. Research into the factors responsible is shifting attention from the protective role of antibodies to that of white blood cells, called killer T lymphocytes, and may revolutionise our approach to producing HIV vaccines.

Though often effective, the antibody arm of our immune system suffers from two limitations. First, each antibody recognises only a small portion of the outer coat of the virus. If the virus changes this key envelope protein, the antibody does not detect it. Secondly, while antibodies are good at mopping up viruses in the bloodstream, they are blind to a virus that has concealed itself inside our cells.

Killer lymphocytes, on the other hand, can recognise many of the different fragments of a virus which appear on the surface of infected cells. T cells active specifically against HIV appear early after exposure to the virus and their levels remain high in people resistant to the disease.

"The correlates of natural immunity may give us an idea of what we should be pursuing", Dr Peggy Johnston, of the US National Institute for Allergy and Infectious Diseases, told a recent Washington meeting on HIV. Such advances may not yet mark the long-awaited dawn, but there is already a discernible lightening of the gloom.

Postscript

In 1986, 227 of the world's leading clinical scientists were asked to predict the state of medicine in the twenty years' time. [See

Chapter 19] Sixty percent thought that we would have a safe and effective vaccine by 2000. Twenty years later, we are still waiting.

One reason is the fast mutation rate of HIV already mentioned. Antibodies that develop against one version of the virus fail to respond when they encounter it again in mutated form. A second reason is that from the outset HIV has existed in several different subtypes, often related to geography. So – to be effective worldwide – either a single vaccine must be effective against many different subtypes, or we will need to give people several different vaccines.

The international AIDS congresses started in Atlanta in 1985, with 2,000 participants. The first I attended was Paris in 1986. By 1991, in Florence, there were 8,000 participants. There had been initial optimism, with evidence that giving HIV-positive people zidovudine (AZT) could slow progression to AIDS and death – but the time gained was on average only six months. And 1991 was a time of growing desperation.

And then in Berlin in 1993, with 14,000 participants, when the theme was "tear down the walls" of discrimination that separate HIV-positive people from others, there was no end to the desperation: the Concorde trial showed no medium- or long-term benefit from starting treatment earlier. And the first trials in which we combined nucleoside analogue drugs failed to improve on single-drug treatment.

In Vancouver in 1996 the atmosphere had been almost miraculously transformed by emerging evidence that combining drugs with *different* mechanisms of action could turn HIV infection from an almost certain death sentence into a chronic illness. As it turned out, we needed three drugs not two; but three was indeed enough to pose HIV a question it could not answer.

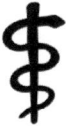

I was once in a pub where the toilets were "Herpes" and "Hispes". You could never joke like that about HIV.

Herpes is a family of viruses, including herpes 1 and 2 and chickenpox (varicella). Herpes strains 1 and 2 are responsible for sores around the mouth and/or genitals: it used to be that one strain was found "below the belt" and one above. With so much oral sex, this distinction no longer applies.

Like chickenpox, which may recur in older age as shingles, herpes 1 and 2 – though dormant for long periods – can always come back, and they may do so frequently if you are unlucky. If you've got it, you've got it for life.

Concern about genital herpes waxes and wanes. Herpes can be inconvenient, annoying, and painful – but (unless you are immunocompromised or infected during birth) it doesn't cause fatal or severe disease. Even so, there were fears of an impending epidemic, and people who wrote about it. Mea culpa.

HERPES SPREAD REACHING EPIDEMIC LEVELS

The Independent September 1995

Unlike true love, herpes lasts forever. And unlike the perfect partner, it is far easier to catch. At least one in eight British women and one in 30 men are infected with the virus that causes genital herpes, according to research conducted at the

Middlesex Hospital last year by a team seeking antibodies to the virus in blood donated for transfusion.

"These figures show that infection is five times more common than we previously thought," says Dr Raj Patel, consultant in genitourinary medicine at the Royal South Hampshire Hospital in Southampton. "We were aware of the people seriously enough affected to seek help, but they represent only about 20 per cent of the total number infected. Given this new evidence, doctors are urgently debating how to reduce the spread of the disease."

Over the past 10 years, genital herpes has been overshadowed by fear of AIDS. But although not fatal, herpes can cause great discomfort, and concern about giving the disease to others can destroy sex lives. Typically, inflammation of part of the genitals is followed by small ulcers which heal over a week or so. The frequency of attacks varies greatly from one person to another, but the disease can recur as often as once a month.

Many people identified by blood test as carrying the virus say they are not aware they have genital herpes. In some, this is probably because the symptoms caused by the disease are slight enough to be misinterpreted as chafing by tight underwear or intercourse. Others have no symptoms at all.

The fact that the disease can be mild is encouraging for some. On the other hand, people who have few problems themselves may cause major problems in others by spreading the disease unwittingly. There is no way of telling how serious herpes will be in a newly infected person. And, once the virus is present, it is there for life.

Dr Larry Corey and colleagues at the University of Washington, in Seattle, recently asked a group of women with herpes to take a swab from their genitals every day for 10 weeks. Sensitive methods of detection showed the virus was frequently present even on days when the women had no symptoms. Doctors have not yet proved that this asymptomatic shedding of virus is sufficient to be infectious, but many believe it is.

"We have known for years that more than half of all herpes transmission occurs from people who have not been diagnosed as having the disease or from people who have no symptoms at the time of intercourse," warns Dr Patel. "This new American research may show why."

Nevertheless, not all recent findings about herpes are gloomy. "It is true that we do not have a pill that will kill the virus stone dead," says Dr Simon Barton, a consultant at London's Chelsea and Westminster Hospital. "But the severity of an attack can be significantly reduced if people start taking the antiviral drug acyclovir as soon as they become aware that a recurrence is imminent. And perhaps a third of them can abort attacks entirely."

Studies have also confirmed that people who suffer more than six herpes episodes per year benefit by taking acyclovir continuously. With such suppressive therapy, up to 90 per cent remain free of attacks over a year. "The original studies involved people with frequent herpes episodes, but anyone whose psychosexual health is appreciably affected by the disease should be offered continuous therapy," says Dr Barton.

There is another potentially exciting side to suppressive therapy. Dr Corey's Seattle labs have discovered that continuous use of acyclovir can reduce the rate at which the virus is shed from the genital tract even during periods between attacks. If this reduction in asymptomatic shedding can be confirmed, and if people carrying the virus can be identified, we may have a way of reducing the spread of the epidemic.

Another possibility is a vaccine. We are familiar with the idea that vaccination prevents people from acquiring an infection. But it seems that vaccines can also boost the immune response of people already infected by the herpes virus, so reducing the severity of the disease. A study published last year in the *Lancet* showed vaccination cut the frequency of herpes episodes by a quarter. New vaccines under development should improve on this figure.

"But the most important goal is to reduce the infectivity of people carrying the herpes virus," says leading vaccine researcher Dr Stephen Straus, of the American National Institutes of Health. It will be some time before we know whether vaccines can achieve that aim, but Dr Straus and colleagues think the strategy worth pursuing.

"At the moment, though, the best advice we can give is that condoms should be used all the time, and not just when there are symptoms of genital herpes," says Dr Patel. "The virus can be transmitted to areas not covered by the condom and spread can occur through oral-genital contact. But condoms are the best option for reducing the risk of disease."

In the United States, some estimates suggest that 45 million people – one in four of the adult population – already carry the herpes virus. This is double the number of 10 years ago. According to Dr Mike Reitano, a New York-based specialist, if we do not soon find an effective way of stopping the spread of herpes, the question of transmission will simply go away – because everyone will have it. The situation in the UK is not yet as serious, but it may become so unless we are able to develop new means of tackling the problem.

Postscript

Many people who became sexually active in the period post the pill but pre HIV are seropositive for one or both herpes strains. Many, though, have never had any symptoms and may never develop them. In writing this piece, I was somewhat taken in by drug company hype. My only defence is that I imparted some sound science along the way.

We now have vaccines effective against chickenpox and its recurrence as shingles. But efforts to prouce a vaccine against genital herpes have not been successful.

Chapter Four

Affairs of the heart

From the Introduction to *Heart Disease: What it is and how it's treated* (written with John Wallwork; Basil Blackwell, Oxford, 1987)...

In our imagination, the heart swells with love, breaks in misery, is strong in the brave, warm in the friendly and cold in the unfeeling. In reality, it is a compact, efficient, tireless and extremely reliable pump. Blood flows in and is forced out. But at times of great emotion we can actually feel the heart move, and perhaps because of this it has come to symbolise so much of human experience and embody life itself.

The heart's chambers, valves and electrical circuits are supreme examples of evolutionary engineering. In an average day the heart beats a hundred thousand times and circulates two thousand gallons of blood – all powered by contraction of the muscle that forms the heart's walls.

Problems can develop through weakened valves and dodgy electrics. But the most common cause is constriction or blockage of the vessels, the coronary arteries, that provide blood to heart muscle itself. It is this that causes a heart attack ...

In the past thirty years, our ability to restore blood flow while heart attacks are happening – and to reduce the risk that they will occur – has revolutionised treatment to an extent unparalleled in any other area of medicine.

That is a big statement. But, with the possible exception of HIV and AIDS, I think it is true. It should not diminish the achievement to say that restoring function to the heart is essentially a matter of emergency plumbing – partly by way of providing new blood vessels to bypass old ones, and partly by way of unblocking those that already exist. This became possible with the advent of thrombolytics – commonly referred to as clot-busting drugs.

The British Cardiac Society was founded in 1922 as the Cardiac Club. In the 1980s, it was still a bow-tied bastion of the old school. In that tradition, members referred to each other by surnames; and in research papers, patients were still called "clinical material".

Flushed with the informality of other medical meetings, I assumed a well-intentioned medical journalist would be welcome at their 1985 annual meeting in Birmingham. But as soon as it became apparent there was a stranger in their midst, there had to be a meeting within the meeting to decide whether I should be asked to leave.

It was the year Desmond Julian took over from Michael Oliver as President; and I'm not sure who was in charge at the time. Whoever it was, he generously encouraged the organizing committee to allow me to stay – on condition that I cleared my reports with speakers. That was a condition I was happy to accept. And it was worthwhile since at that meeting I learned a great deal of what was to revolutionise cardiology over the next decade.

FOUR HOURS TO BEAT THE CLOT

The Guardian May 1985

New techniques to treat heart attacks have been tried in Holland but are far from routine in British hospitals.

A foreign correspondent in medicine

Unpublished results of a Dutch study show that heart attack patients are significantly less likely to die if they have an injection of streptokinase within a few hours of the onset of symptoms. The trial, which was co-ordinated in Rotterdam and took four years to conduct, showed that streptokinase not only reduced the death rate from heart attack but also resulted in less loss of heart muscle and heart function in those who survived.

Susceptibility to a heart attack builds over many years as the blood vessels supplying the heart muscle become narrowed by fatty deposits laid down along their walls. But the event that precipitates the attack is a sudden blockage of the narrowed artery by a blood clot. Streptokinase dissolves the clot, blood supply is restored, and as a result less heart muscle dies from lack of oxygen.

The five Dutch hospitals which took part in the study randomised more than five hundred heart attack patients to either standard treatment or to standard treatment plus streptokinase. Within the following month, 31 of the 266 people not given streptokinase died. Of those receiving the clot dissolving enzyme, there were only 14 deaths among the same number of patients. Mortality was reduced from 12% to 5%.

That represents a dramatic advance. David de Bono, who works on clot-busting drugs at the Edinburgh Royal Infirmary, talks of a future in which drugs will be like "fire and forget" missiles that find the clot and destroy it[1]. But there are a number of caveats. First, the drugs in the Dutch

---

[1] This was only three years after the formidable capability of missiles such as the Exocet had been demonstrated during the Falklands War.

trial were administered directly into the coronary arteries of patients in highly specialised hospital units.

Secondly, the patients who benefited were on average given the drugs within two hours of first experiencing chest pain. It is thought that the window of opportunity closes after around four hours. Given the race against time, if clot busting drugs are to become routine they will have to be given outside hospital, and they will have to work when given by intravenous injection.

It is also important to understand that treating heart attack successfully is a package deal. Chemically dissolving the clot itself is only a first step. More often than not, it must be followed by mechanical intervention to reverse the narrowing that gave the clot the opportunity to block the artery in the first place.

The rise of balloons

Fortunately, new ways of restoring the diameter of vital coronary arteries (techniques called angioplasty) also offer fresh hope for the heart.

One procedure involves inflating a tiny balloon inside the partly obstructed artery, squeezing cholesterol-laden plaque back into the blood vessel wall. Balloon angioplasty is becoming routine in the US, where there have been 65,000 such procedures, and is being piloted in specialised UK hospitals.

A fine tube (or catheter) is inserted into a major blood vessel in the patient's arm or leg and gently eased towards the heart. In a virtuoso feat of navigation, it is manoeuvred into the 2–3mm wide opening of a coronary artery and along its length until the inflatable section sits astride the narrowing.

Liquid is then pumped into the balloon until it is fully

expanded. Inflation usually lasts 15–30 seconds, using a pressure equivalent to four or five atmospheres – much the same force as when you stamp on an acorn. And the effect is similar. In both cases, the object is squashed flat. But, while squashing an acorn is usually without risk, coronary angioplasty is not. It requires daring as well as dexterity. There is a danger that the coronary artery may split under too much pressure, or that small pieces of plaque will break off and travel round the body, becoming lodged in still smaller blood vessels such as those in the brain.

As David de Bono says, "The operation is performed under heavy sedation, and not just of the patient". But balloon angioplasty can be highly effective and requires only short hospital admission. It is also becoming a routine method of helping people with chronic chest pain (angina) caused by coronary artery narrowing and is spawning a new species of "interventional" cardiologists who now have something to match the prowess of their cardiac surgeon colleagues.

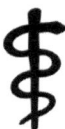

Hope springs eternal: the coronary stent

The Guardian January 1988

The careful positioning of a flexible, coiled spring inside the heart's blood vessels is helping doctors to

keep open crucial coronary arteries and so preserve the supply of blood to heart muscle. The stainless steel coil, developed in Switzerland, is now under trial at the National Heart Hospital in London.

Clots that form during a heart attack can often be cleared by pushing a catheter through them and then inflating a tiny balloon – a technique called angioplasty – to push the sides of the artery apart. But blood vessels are delicate and may respond to the insult by closing up altogether once the balloon is removed or over the next few weeks. Hence the need for a mechanical means of safeguarding the passage of blood.

Early results suggest that use of the steel coil – two strands of wire woven into a double helix about 2cm long and 3–4mm in diameter – is highly promising.

Coils are positioned in the coronary artery in a compressed state using a catheter similar to the one used in balloon angioplasty. The membrane keeping the spring compressed is then withdrawn allowing the helix to expand. The coil – termed a stent – was first used in Toulouse, in 1986. Since then, 80 have been used, mostly at the University Hospital of Lausanne. In ten patients, the spring provoked a blockage, which was successfully cleared in all but four. Fourteen patients have experienced the development of a blockage over a longer period.

Five patients died, but two were in the process of having a heart attack when the spring was used as a last resort. In only two cases was the stent the cause of death. In the great majority the new device has been used without adverse effects.

Dr Anthony Rickards, of the National Heart Hospital, was the first cardiologist in the UK to implant a stent. He emphasised: "We're still feeling our way with this device. It is very experimental and its tendency to cause clots in the early stages is undoubtedly a worry at the moment. But a new version about to come out has a coating that allows the anticoagulant drug heparin to be actually bonded to the coil."

Postscript

The majority of stents implanted today have a coating on the coil which gradually releases a drug to reduce the risk of clot formation, much as Dr Rickards envisaged in 1988. Regarded as one of the best cardiologists of his generation, he died in 2004. With many thousands of stents implanted each year in the UK (and two million worldwide), coronary stenting is now commonplace as a treatment following a heart attack and to prevent such attacks in people with angina.

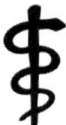

Post-mortem examination of young US soldiers killed in Korea first alerted the medical profession to the widespread and early onset of coronary artery disease. For decades afterwards, the age-related silting up of these crucial blood vessels seemed an inevitable part of the Western way of life, and death. Highly committed individuals might slow the worsening of atheroma by exercise and substantial changes to diet. But, at the population level, it seemed that nothing much could be done. Then came statins.

According to the Nuffield Department of Population Health in Oxford, statins – like or loathe them – are the most commonly prescribed class of medicine in the UK, and for good reason. They save lives, and they don't cause many side-effects. There was a time, though, when they were not in virtually every elderly person's pill box but a novel idea that had barely been tested.

THE DAWN OF STATINS

Pharmacy Update April 1987

Between half and two-thirds of the 100–150grams of cholesterol that we all contain is made by our own bodies, mostly in the liver. If we want to lower cholesterol levels, switching this production off is a sensible idea; and the first drugs based on this principle should soon become available.

Clinical trials in the USA, Canada and Finland show the fungal metabolite lovastatin – the first of this new class of drugs – is safe and effective. More than a thousand patients have now been treated for up to four years. Typically, they experience a 30% fall in plasma total cholesterol, a 40% decrease in the highly atherogenic low-density lipoprotein (LDL) cholesterol fraction, and an increase of 5–10% in protective HDL.

Dr Roger Illingworth, from Portland, Oregon, has the greatest experience of the new agent. Speaking at a conference in Helsinki he confirmed that long-term use of the drug has a sustained cholesterol-reducing effect.

Lovastatin works by inhibiting a key enzyme involved in the body's synthesis of choleseterol. Since cholesterol – although playing a villain's part in clogging up coronary arteries – is also a vital component of cell walls and steroid hormones, the body reacts to a reduction in its production by increasing the extraction of cholesterol from blood plasma. The meeting heard that reducing plasma cholesterol levels by

10% – whether by drugs or diet – produces a 15% reduction in coronary heart disease after two years.

TURNING BACK THE CLOCK

Medical Monitor March 1990

Reducing coronary mortality is one thing. Reversing the underlying disease is altogether more challenging, and the idea that something might be done gained traction only gradually. But, in 1987, David Blankenhorn and colleagues from the University of Southern California reported results from a landmark trial in which men who had already had bypass grafts for coronary artery disease were randomised to placebo or two cholesterol-lowering drugs.

Two years of treatment halved levels of LDL-cholesterol and increased HDL levels by 37%. The really striking finding, though, was that the narrowing in coronary arteries became measurably less with time in 16% of men on drug treatment. This compared with 2% in the group taking placebo pills. Well over half the actively treated men showed either regression of atheroma or stable disease. Time on their coronary clock had stopped ticking away.

More than a hundred patients in this study have now been followed for four years. Details of their condition were given at the recent [1989] New Orleans meeting of the American Heart Association. Compared with the control group, drug therapy more than halved the rate of progression of coronary artery disease; and the proportion of patients with documented regression was almost three times that among men randomised to placebo.

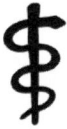

Engine and gearbox: another Cambridge first?

World Medicine March 1983

Surgeons at Papworth Hospital, Cambridge, are close to performing Britain's first heart-lung transplant – a little like replacing engine and gearbox, "you have a matched unit".

The simultaneous removal and replacement of a heart plus both lungs is a formidable procedure. But it is the only treatment to offer hope in many cases of advanced heart and lung disease. And there is a clear logic. If you are going to transplant both lungs, then – provided it will benefit the patient – you may as well take the heart as well. It is a little like replacing engine and gearbox together, say surgeons.

Procedures have been refined in primates to the point where the necessary techniques are well understood. New techniques of immune suppression offer a good prospect of controlling rejection. And, most important of all, surgeons at Stanford in the United States have proved the operation works in man.

Pioneered by Bruce Reitz, working under the direction of Norman Shumway, there have now been eleven heart-lung transplants in California. Seven of the patients are alive. The longest survivor, Mary, had her operation in March 1981, and long ago returned to her job as an editor.

The second transplant, on a 30-year-old man, was also a success. Chuck had been a blue baby, and a blue adult, almost totally unable to exercise. Since the operation he has learned to swim and for the first time in his life can ride a bicycle.

In the UK, the Papworth group has two kinds of recipient in mind. The first is people with primary lung disorders such as pulmonary hypertension, where most of the damage is to the lungs, but the heart may also be involved. The second group has primary heart problems, but the associated lung condition is serious enough to make a straightforward heart transplant impractical.

A promise fulfilled

Both groups are relatively young, and neither can be much helped by conventional medical or surgical treatment. Many patients are terminally ill; in most, the quality of any remaining life is poor.

Although corrective surgery is possible in many cases of congenital heart disease, there is a group of patients with particularly complex problems. These are the people who as babies received palliative treatment in the hope that in the future something better would come along. Now many of them are reaching adolescence, and they are still waiting. For them, a heart-lung transplant would be a promise fulfilled.

But even with such severe problems, need the solution always be as radical as a heart lung transplant? Would it not be enough to replace a single lung? Experience suggests not: if you are going to transplant one lung, you may as well

Engine and gearbox: another Cambridge first?

transplant both. Of the 35 patients who have had unilateral lung replacements, only three survived thirty days and none survived a year. Retaining one of the original damaged lungs increases the chances of cross-infection and may cause imbalance in ventilation.

And if you are going to transplant both lungs, it makes sense to take the heart as well. While more difficult in some respects than heart transplantation, the heart-lung operation is easier in others. Taking the damaged organs out of the recipient takes longer. But the reconnection of donor organs requires only three long sutures instead of four.

As well as the relative ease of reconnection, the presence of a transplanted heart has one notable advantage. It enables tissue rejection to be detected early using a biopsy method which is not possible with lung tissue alone. This allows immunosuppression to be tailored to the exact condition of the transplant. Episodes of rejection can be aborted, and the risk of over-suppression during lulls in the immune response is reduced.

The introduction of cyclosporin A, which the Papworth group started to use in March 1982, has reduced the frequency of rejection. By replacing steroids, it meant fewer problems of infection, and less worry that immunosuppression will interfere with healing.

Problems with the availability and preservation of donor organs are the main reasons the programme has not already started. John Wallwork, Papworth surgeon and Transplant Service Director, compared the position to that of people building a lifeboat. They can see others drowning but are aware there are still holes in the hull. Set out too soon and the rescue boat sinks, however good its design.

Postscript

At the time of writing, Papworth Hospital was a rambling ex-tuberculosis sanatorium in the village of Papworth Everard, twelve miles west of Cambridge, but it was already a centre of exceptional achievement. Terence English had performed the first successful UK heart transplant there in 1979. The recipient, Keith Castle, survived more than five years.

As it turned out, Papworth was not the first UK hospital to perform a heart-lung transplant. That was carried out at Harefield Hospital in December 1983. But the recipient, Swedish journalist Lars Ljungberg (sic) died 13 days later. Papworth performed the first *successful* heart-lung transplant in 1984.

There are now around ten heart-lung transplants each year in the UK. This compares with roughly two hundred heart transplants, so the heart-lung procedure never became a major form of heart-related transplant, as John Wallwork envisaged it might. But it can be a very successful operation. Around half those who have the transplant survive for at least five years.

In 2018, Papworth Hospital moved to the Addenbrooke's campus in Cambridge and was given the designation "Royal".

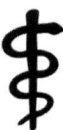

Defibrillators are now commonplace in community centres and even in country phone boxes. But there was a time when they were a life-saving innovation.

For the Man Having a Heart Attack on Platform 1

The Guardian September 1987

Though long past the age of steam, railway stations are still the scene of much huffing and puffing as passengers scramble for trains. British Transport Police at London's Victoria Station are notified each year of around thirty sudden deaths – most caused by heart attacks that lead to fatal arrhythmias.

To Douglas Chamberlain, a consultant cardiologist in Brighton, at the other end of the line from Victoria, the obvious solution was to install defibrillators capable of shocking the heart back into healthy rhythm. Funded by £20,000 from the British Heart Foundation, he was the prime mover behind the deployment of these devices at Victoria and Brighton stations in 1987. In his capacity as cardiology adviser to British Caledonian, he had already had the airline provide defibrillators on long-haul flights.

In most heart attacks, a clot obstructs a narrowed coronary artery cutting off the blood supply to an area of heart muscle which dies over a period of hours. There is pain, and the heart's pumping capacity is reduced, but it carries on.

In a minority of cases, the heart's electrical control system is affected and the result is uncoordinated muscular contractions – or fibrillation – which effectively ends all pumping of blood, in which case death occurs within minutes. Hence the importance of having at close hand devices that can restore normal rhythm.

Ambulances are traditionally white taxis with whirling lights, good for ferrying heart attack victims to hospital but of less help than they could be along the way. This year [1987], the government recognised the need for ambulance personnel to be trained in the use of life-saving intravenous drugs and defibrillators.

Action stations for defibrillators

American cities show what can be done. In Seattle, where firemen double as emergency medical technicians trained in advanced life support, the average time between someone collapsing from a heart attack and the delivery of a defibrillating shock is eight minutes. More than half of the patients treated reach hospital alive, and one in four survives to be discharged.

In Northern Ireland, pre-hospital coronary care is also well developed. Specialist ambulances equipped with defibrillators reach Belfast's collapsed coronary cases in ten minutes. And it is routine for rural GPs to carry a defibrillator in their cars. This practice may soon be widespread on the mainland.

Most sudden heart attack deaths occur like a bolt from the blue. But some people are known to be at high risk of fibrillation because their heart is clearly damaged, usually as the result of a previous heart attack. There is no reason in principle why these people should not have a defibrillator as a piece of household furniture. The practical objection to DIY defibrillation is of course that not all cases of collapse are due to a defibrillating heart; and the casualty's spouse is probably not best placed to judge. One way around the problem is the automatic detector-defibrillator, which lets the machine's disinterested logic decide.

More radical is to have defibrillators that can be implanted in the patient like a pacemaker. Weighing about 300 grams and no larger than a Swan Vestas matchbox, the device continuously monitors cardiac rhythm and delivers a corrective shock when life-threatening arrhythmias are detected. Since 1984, when Edgar Sowton placed one in a Guy's Hospital patient, eight implanted defibrillators have been used in Britain, at almost £10,000 apiece.

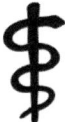

SNAKE VENOM IS AN ACE SOLUTION

The Guardian May 1989

Study of the American pit viper led to a new class of drug offering hope for a growing number of diseases of the heart and blood vessels.

About one in three people with diabetes who are dependent on insulin eventually develops kidney failure. Hope that this problem can be delayed, perhaps even prevented, comes from the latest research into a new class of drugs called ACE inhibitors which owes its discovery to research on the venom of the South American pit viper.

A foreign correspondent in medicine

ACE inhibitors are likely to prove as significant to modern medicine as the Nobel prize-winning discovery of beta blockers. They are already used to treat high blood pressure and heart failure and may prove to have a role in brain problems such as Alzheimer's disease.

However broad their eventual application, much current interest is focused on the potential of ACE inhibitors to decrease the long-term kidney damage caused by diabetes.

People with adult-onset diabetes tend to have high blood pressure at the time their diabetes is diagnosed. But diabetics dependent on insulin develop the condition in the course of their disease – at roughly the same time as kidney damage becomes apparent.

This close association is certainly not accident. It was once thought that the kidney problems caused raised blood pressure. But many doctors now argue that the reverse is true. This is an important change in thinking because, while we have no established way of reversing kidney damage, we have well-tried means of reducing blood pressure.

Losing weight, cutting down on salt and taking exercise are important ways of doing this without resorting to drugs. But full control of high blood pressure usually requires pharmacological intervention.

Hans-Henrik Parving, in Denmark, was one of the first doctors to urge aggressive treatment of high blood pressure in diabetics with established kidney disease. He showed convincingly that effective control of hypertension slowed the decline in kidney function. Before treatment, his patients were on course for dialysis or transplant within seven years. At the present rate of deterioration, it looks as if their kidneys will hold out for at least three times that long.

One of the main signs of kidney damage is finding protein in the urine. Its presence shows that the kidneys are sufficiently "leaky" to allow large molecules through. The problem can be detected by dipping a protein-sensitive strip in the urine. Using more sophisticated instruments, it is possible to detect far lower levels of protein – a condition called microalbuminuria. In itself, this is not harmful, but it is certainly a marker of early kidney damage.

Doctors had established that reducing high blood pressure helped patients with obvious kidney damage. The next question was whether they should give drugs to diabetics with normal blood pressure and only slight signs of kidney damage in the hope of catching the condition early, and perhaps of preventing it.

Certain scientists, among them Barry Brenner from Harvard, believe that pressure within the filtering units (or glomeruli) of the kidney may be damagingly high even when blood pressure within the rest of the circulation is normal. This is where the ACE inhibitors become important, as they may have a specific effect in reducing high pressures within the glomeruli.

Much of the work supporting this idea has come from animal experiments. But hopeful evidence in patients is beginning to emerge. Apparently, ACE inhibitors do reduce the amount of protein in the urine at doses which do not lower the normal blood pressure in the rest of the circulation.

Dr Parving has demonstrated this in a small group of patients in Denmark. Research from Michel Marré in Paris, who has also used an ACE inhibitor in diabetic patients with microalbuminuria but normal blood pressure, shows the same effect. If these early results are confirmed, doctors may begin to prescribe ACE inhibitors to diabetics with normal blood pressure but early signs of kidney problems.

As well as their potential in reducing the complications of diabetes, ACE inhibitors may have a role in brain disease. One of the most surprising findings to emerge from a meeting on ACE inhibitors held last year [1988] in Cannes was that memory deficits in rats could be reversed. This work, from the University of Heidelberg, has now been reinforced by animal studies from the Bradford University School of Pharmacy.

Professor Brenda Costall told a recent London meeting that learning impairment caused by drugs and by damage to certain areas of the brain can be countered by giving a new ACE inhibitor specifically targeted at the central nervous system. Although it is unwise to extrapolate from these early results, Professor Costall is impressed by the similarities between her models of memory deficits in animals and Alzheimer's disease. The first results of clinical trials using ACE inhibitors in patients with age-related deterioration in memory should be released later this year.

Postscript

An ACE inhibitor generally features in the top-five lists of the world's most frequently prescribed medicines. ACE inhibitors have become a mainstay of cardiovascular medicine, central to the treatment of people with hypertension or heart failure and for those who have had a heart attack. NICE also recommends that people with type I or type 2 diabetes and microalbuminuria should take an ACE inhibitor, even if they do not have high blood pressure, since these drugs slow the progression of kidney disease.

Snake venom is an ACE solution

Around ten years ago, evidence was published suggesting that ACE inhibitors might slow cognitive decline in the elderly, but to date this has never been convincing enough for regulatory authorities to allow them to be prescribed for this reason.

Chapter Five

Murder most foul, or murder most foolish?

World Medicine January 1984

Surgeon Paul Vickers was jailed in 1981 for murdering his wife with the brain cancer drug CCNU. But there is argument about the evidence. Interviewed in Wakefield jail, Vickers gave an account that was bizarre but just about believable.

Consultant orthopaedic surgeon Paul Vickers repeatedly gives his schizophrenic and crippled wife Margaret the rare, dangerous and undetectable drug CCNU, without any monitoring of its likely toxic effects on her bone marrow, and with no evidence she has cancer. The prescriptions, cashed in a London chemist by his mistress, Pamela Collison, are made out to a series of false names.

Within five months, Margaret Vickers is in hospital. Her blood platelet and white cell counts are at rock bottom. Within nine months, she dies of aplastic anaemia. At no point during her critical illness does her husband mention the CCNU (also known as lomustine) to anyone caring for his wife, though he cannot have failed to see its relevance. Indecently soon after Margaret's death in June 1979, Pamela Collison arranges a date for their marriage. It never takes

Murder most foul, or murder most foolish?

place, but the motive and means for murder could hardly seem more plain.

When it came to the trial of Vickers and Collison, the main facts of the case, including CCNU as a cause of death, were not really disputed. After five weeks, twelve good citizens of Teesside took only five hours to agree unanimously on Vickers' guilt. They took another fifteen minutes to find Collison, whom the crowd later hissed and booed, not guilty by a majority verdict.

Presiding, the Honourable Mr Justice Boreham (fresh from the trial of the Yorkshire Ripper) said that man's inhumanity had plumbed new depths and recommended at least seventeen years. Collison was whisked off for twelve days of interrogation by the *News of the World*. And everyone else went home – except for Paul Vickers, who went to Wakefield jail, where he spends his time writing letters about his case and preparing engineering drawings for the prison workshop. Many would consider him fortunate. The only other doctors convicted this century of murdering their wives, Crippen and Ruxton, ended on the wrong end of a rope.

The Vickers case excites the prurient imagination. There were allegations that Collison started the affair by following Vickers into his hotel room and taking off all her clothes. One of Vickers' letters to her spoke of his need for someone to be "a wife, mistress and whore". Vickers said that he had noticed scars on Collison's loin which she claimed came from being whipped. And all through the trial there was the tantalising prospect that the web of sexual revelations might entangle the national political figures with whom Collison had also associated.

There was the spectacle in court of a big fish out of water

and being gutted. Vickers was not only approved as a prospective Tory candidate for the European Parliament, he had served on the General Medical Council and still sat in judgment on his fellows as a member of the central ethical committee of the British Medical Association.

If the spectacle of the whole sordid, melodramatic mess was compelling, so too were the facts of the case. It takes a leap of imagination to countenance any explanation other than cunning, cold-blooded murder.

But there is an alternative account, not fully reported before. Paul Vickers does not come out well. He is extraordinarily stupid, and probably almost as deluded as his schizophrenic wife, who at one point thought she had transistor radios in her teeth. He is also weak – something like the defence counsel's description of a "collapsed blancmange of a man". But he is not a murderer.

One of the keys to understanding this account is the peculiar relationship Vickers had with his wife, both as husband and as virtual sole physician. For seventeen years, he was her medical adviser on everything, including her schizophrenia. He seems to have been both distrustful of his colleagues' ability to treat her, and arrogant about his own. Suspicion may have stemmed from a period before their marriage when psychiatrists tried to get him to persuade an unwilling Margaret to have ECT. She too deeply distrusted other doctors.

Whatever the reasons, over almost two decades, Vickers had become used to prescribing drugs for his wife on his own responsibility, and Margaret had become used to taking them. He had even prescribed for her using the name of one of his mistresses as the patient – presumably because he did not want it widely known either that his wife was ill or that he was treating her. This "secret of schizophrenia" was one for them alone to share.

Against this background, it is not quite so sinister that the CCNU prescriptions were in false names. It strengthens Vickers' claim that, although he wrote out the first prescription correctly, he saw nothing morally wrong in using false names when Collison protested embarrassment at having to collect the drugs as Margaret Vickers.

The crucial question, though, is why he should want to give Margaret CCNU – if not to poison her.

Paul Vickers' version of events is that Margaret said she had a brain tumour and he believed her. There is no independent evidence that she said anything of the sort. But there are two reasons for thinking she might have done. One is that it is not uncommon for people with schizophrenia to look for some organic reason for their disease. The other is that a friend of the Vickers', whose symptoms resembled Margaret's, had recently had a brain tumour diagnosed.

There is also the fact that Vickers too had consistently looked for organic pathology as a more acceptable explanation for his wife's condition. When Margaret was briefly certified in 1962, he had her investigated for a thyroid condition. He even persisted in prescribing for thyrotoxicosis after investigation had shown she did not have the condition.

Assuming for a moment that his wife did say she had a tumour, and that Vickers thought it possible, why in the name of all that is sacred in diagnostics did he not get an expert neurologist's opinion? It takes more than shared suspicion of other doctors to account for this astonishing lapse in professional standards: we have to accept the existence of a shared delusion. But could even seventeen years of living with a person with schizophrenia have caused some of Vickers' ideas to become as divorced from reality as those of his wife?

Psychiatric evidence at the trial was that Vickers' life had become compartmentalised. Although behaving normally as a doctor outside the home, it is just about believable that he could have had totally irrational ideas of diagnosis and treatment in the domestic context when dealing with his wife.

The theory of *folie à deux* was put at the trial by Dr Renton, and accepted as tenable by Dr Hawkins. Although the prosecution had access to psychiatrists, they never sought to rebut it. This omission could — perhaps should — have been referred to in the judge's summing up. It was not. And the Vickers trial is one of several in the past few years (another being that of Peter Sutcliffe, where the judge and prosecution team were the same as for Vickers) in which psychiatric testimony seemed to have little impact.

There is evidence, from what Vickers told doctors at the time Margaret was admitted to hospital in 1979, that he uncritically accepted his wife's accounts of her medical condition. She had told him of a three-month illness in the autumn, and he passed the information on as though he had seen it too. It is fairly clear from the diary of Margaret's activities at the time, and from people who saw her, that she was not in fact in poor health.

That is slim evidence of shared delusion, but it is there. There is certainly evidence that Vickers' mental state could be odd. Robert Souhami, an oncologist with experience of CCNU, remembers Vickers from before the trial. "His mind was a mush about events surrounding his wife's death," Dr Souhami recalls. "Though he could be quite rational about other things."

But there is great difficulty in understanding Vickers' failure to mention CCNU when his wife was in hospital and so in the medical context in which he functioned competently. Take the *deux* away from the *folie,* and it fades.

Vickers' account here – and it is difficult to credit – is that he did not immediately realise the significance of CCNU. It was not until a colleague phoned to ask if he had X-ray equipment at home, with the idea that Margaret might have caused the bone marrow damage by X-raying herself, that he saw the link between cancer treatment and his wife's condition. Even with this realisation, there was no need to say anything. To have admitted the CCNU "therapy" would have made them both seem ludicrous. He would have risked being struck off; and it would not have helped Margaret's recovery, which was progressing quite well at the time.

The other major problem in the defence is how to account for the fact that prescriptions for CCNU continued to be written, and dispensed, in the months between Margaret's partial recovery and her ultimate death. It looks very much as if, having failed to kill her at the first attempt, more of the drug was obtained to finish the job.

The explanation offered is blackmail. In an effort to maintain her hold on Vickers, Pamela Collison is alleged to have insisted that he continue to write prescriptions. If he did not oblige, she threatened to reveal that he had already been obtaining drugs under false names.

That is plausible when Collison's previous conduct is taken into account. There is good evidence that she was capable of extreme vindictiveness. In court, publisher David Croom told of how Collison had hounded him from London to a wedding in Edinburgh where, in public, she accused him loudly, and apparently falsely, of making her pregnant. On other occasions, she was said to have besieged his flat, and attacked him with a knife. According to Vickers, Collison had also spread the story that a previous lover was the Yorkshire Ripper, and it is known the man concerned was questioned by the police.

All this stupidity, delusion and persecution is pretty unlikely, but it is possible. The main reason for giving it some credence is that there are also important oddities about the conclusion – at first sight so obvious – that Vickers was simply poisoning his wife.

The Vickers house was choc-a-bloc with drugs, some samples and some prescribed, many kept in a cocktail cabinet. Margaret was used to taking between two and four capsules a day on her husband's sole advice. She was prone to depression, so a suicide attempt would not have been unlikely. If Vickers wanted to kill her, why did he not simply give her an overdose of the sleeping pills and tranquillisers that were so abundant. He might have been criticised for leaving drugs about, but he would not have been suspected of murder.

Secondly, CCNU would be a tricky drug to use as a poison. Because it was new, unusual and dangerous, careful records were kept of who prescribed it. CCNU was available on private prescription only from John Bell and Croyden of London's Wigmore Street. Details were phoned through to the suppliers, Lundbeck, before each prescription was dispensed. It was like signing the Poisons Register. In the two and a half years after the introduction of CCNU, only 33 private prescriptions were filled; 13 were for Vickers. There was an obvious possibility that his use of it would be queried. An alert marketing manager would have sent a rep straight up the A1 to see how such a regular customer was getting on. Given that he was an orthopaedic surgeon, Vickers would have had some smart explaining to do.

Even if he had decided to go to the extraordinary lengths of using CCNU to murder his wife, why did Vickers administer it in small, regular amounts? The regime he prescribed was eccentric, but in total exposure it probably amounted to no more than the recommended therapeutic dose of five capsules every six to eight weeks. Why did he not give a massive overdose at the start and save his wife a lingering death and himself a lot of trouble?

Her death would have been attributed to naturally occurring aplastic anaemia with sudden onset. No-one would have considered looking for evidence of CCNU, and, anyway, all traces of the drug would have disappeared during the four to six weeks required for it to destroy bone marrow.

The third reason for doubting the prosecution case concerns motive. According to Vickers' account, his infatuation with Collison was well over by the time he started to give his wife CCNU. The Crown argued that the torrid and conspiratorial letters the lovers exchanged were spread monthly over something like two years. Vickers assigned the letters, none of which is dated, to an early and short-lived period of lust.

Postscript

Paul Vickers twice appealed against conviction – in 1983 and again in 1994 – and twice had his appeal rejected.

Chapter Six

Beauty and the bombs

World Medicine May 1984

GPs in Northern Ireland have deeply troubling accounts of the violence being inflicted on their communities.

From the sitting room of Patrick Ward's house, on a clear day, you can see the Mourne mountains. You can also see the puffs of smoke when bombs explode in the border town of Newry, two miles away in the valley. For a doctor, that is useful warning your services will once again be needed.

In the fifteen years since the latest violence began, there have been 235 killings in South Armagh and South Down: 121 civilians among the dead. Only two of the slaughtered were decent old-fashioned murders. The rest were executions, revenge killings, "own goals" from premature explosions, victims of indiscriminate bombings and butchery, casualties in the "war" on the security forces.

For Patrick Ward, this means repeatedly establishing the facts of violent death; once, in the case of a booby-trapped body, with the aid of powerful binoculars. But it is not just the gruesome formalities. Thirty-eight patients on his own general practice list have been killed. And there is the aftermath of grief and bitterness to palliate as best he can.

I went with him on a depressing half-hour drive along

the lanes around Bessbrook. We passed the scenes of 18 murders – the most horrific near Kingsmill, where men returning from work were taken out of their minibus and shot. Dr Ward recalls that evening in January 1976. The day before, three local men had been killed, and there was intimation of revenge.

"People spoke in whispers, and surgery attendances were very sparse. I had a call to do after surgery, but when I drove out to the area my sixth sense advised me it could wait until the following day. It was perhaps fortunate that I made the decision to turn the car a short distance out of Bessbrook.

"I arrived home to receive a telephone call to attend a patient suffering from shock. When I asked the cause, I was told he'd come home after all his pals had been shot dead. My patient told me that at first he thought he was the intended victim (as the only Catholic there), and two of his friends had held his hands and told him not to identify himself.

"I went to the hospital, feeling the bodies would be brought there, but was told to go to the scene. I drove back to find ten men lying dead. As I picked my way, slipping on the blood on the road, from man to man, I was able to identify every one. Eight were my own patients. It was the worst village disaster since Aberfan."

Richard Dorman, one of five GPs in the border town of Keady, was on call the evening of the Darkley killings last year [1983], when worshippers in a mission hall were raked with machine-gun fire.

"It had been a quiet Sunday. There was a car accident in the town, and an injured girl sent off to Craigavon with a lacerated foot. Otherwise, nothing. At 6.25 I got a call to a shooting. I'd only been to one before. That was at a pub in town. A clean entry wound through one eye, the man obviously dead.

"I drove like the hammer two miles up the road. When I got to the hall it was very quiet. There were cars parked outside, but I wondered if I was in the right place. When I walked in there were two men lying dead, crumpled together. One of them had a bad wound in the head, an exit wound taking most of the brain with it. The other had bullet wounds in the neck. There was a man in the doorway telling me he'd been hurt badly. Then I realised there were six or more in the hall, and another man dead. Though no-one was screaming, it was mayhem.

"I checked for acute problems, sent for another doctor (it was my father who came), and went back to the man in the doorway with the abdominal wound. He was going into shock and needed a drip straightaway.

"There was a girl bleeding from her nose. It seemed slight. I told her just to keep pressure on it. Later it turned out a bullet had ricocheted round her sinuses and was lodged there. Another girl was bleeding from her elbow, which she was holding. It was shattered. But she wasn't aware there was a bullet in her side and hadn't lifted up her arm to see.

"By 7.30, most of the patients were away, and no-one who left the hall alive died later. The most difficult part came then – certifying the three men dead. I wanted to be absolutely sure I'd got the identification right because I had to go and tell their wives."

Back in Belfast, Joe Hendron is also in the front line. The Albert Street health centre, off the Falls Road, is fortified like a barracks. It faces the surrounding housing estates with windowless grey and wire-topped walls.

"Most of our patients are unemployed – 80% around the Divis Flats," he says. "But on top of the poverty you have 'the troubles'. There is intimidation from the paramilitary organisations, and hoods and gangsters of all shapes and sizes. When there is a shooting there are searches by the security forces, and these are resented.

"Because of this, the whole quality of life is different from other deprived areas. The result is depressive illness and apathy. But it's not a depression drugs can help. And I don't refer people to psychiatrists. A call to the housing executive or the social security office can be far more use."

Joe Hendron is a man who mixes medicine and politics. He is an SDLP city councillor and fought the Westminster seat, losing to Gerry Adams. Threatened with assassination by both Republican and Loyalist sides, he checks the wheel arches of his car every morning for bombs.

"It becomes a way of life," he says. "I was once held in a house for five hours with a gun to my head while my car was used, as it was termed, 'to transfer personnel from A to B'. I could have a bodyguard, but wouldn't want to put a policeman in danger."

In the tangled bloody mess that is much of Northern Ireland, doctors pass, most of the time, as neutrals. Where the segregation of communities allows, practices have both Protestant and Catholic personnel and patients. But in a country where religion is the basis of social classification, doctors cannot always avoid being labeled.

Raymond Shearer is a GP on the Springfield Road, where

he is close to the RUC barracks that is subject to the occasional "wee rocket attack". He remembers having to do a house call for a Protestant doctor who could not visit a Catholic patient across the street from his surgery because of threats to his safety. In these circumstances, doctors take pains to retain their neutrality by scrupulous fairness. Joe Hendron, who played an important part in revealing "non-accidental injuries" during interrogations at the Castlereagh barracks, is keen to point out that for the majority of police he has nothing but respect.

Doctors adhere strictly to two principles. These are aimed at preserving life, not least their own, as well as being ethical imperatives. First, someone who is ill has to be treated, whoever they are and whatever they have done. Second, what a doctor may know about the activities of his patients is no-one else's business. As Raymond Shearer told me, "The police have a job to do, and so have doctors. To make doctors policemen would put them in an impossible position."

Postscript

At the third attempt, in 1992, Joe Hendron took the Westminster seat of West Belfast from Sinn Féin President Gerry Adams, though Adams regained it five years later. Dr Hendron recently survived being knocked down by a white van.

The Dormans' practice in Keady was both cross-generational and cross-border, and impressive on both counts. After a house call to a patient who lived in a remote caravan, I was taken into the Republic on an unmarked road for what I was promised would be an excellent pint of Guinness. And so it was. "Why are you not having one?" I asked. "Because it's Lent," Dr Dorman replied.

Chapter Seven

Being male means being mortal

SPOTLIGHT ON MEN'S HEALTH

The Independent January 1996

Maybe men ignore warning signs because they have less emotional involvement with their bodies. Or perhaps taking on the sick role conflicts with society's stereotype of male behaviour.

When Lewisham's first Well Man clinic opened a year ago [1995], the provision of free condoms was the lead item in leaflets advertising the service. The offer of a general health check, thought to be something of a turn-off for men, was well down the list. But the hundred or so men who attended the Friday evening clinic over its first six months have brought the idea of a personal MOT to the top of the publicity agenda.

The Lewisham experience shows that some men are not averse to the kind of check-up long familiar to women. Nevertheless, it is a telling point that the Well Man clinic was established as a result of pressure from women.

"We run large Well Woman clinics," says Lindy Bashford, manager of the Lewisham *Open for Men* initiative. "We found women saying they wished something similar was available for their partners, who they felt wouldn't see a doctor until they were actually ill. In response we closed an under-utilised family-planning session and diverted money into the Well Man service."

The men of Lewisham are privileged. Their clinic is one of only five in the country. And this is despite the fact that the Government's document on the state of the public health, published four years ago, identified reduction of illness among men as a national priority.

A James Dean attitude to self-preservation

Men have the advantage of birth: there are 105 boys born to every 100 girls. From then on, the survival stakes are firmly stacked against them. Birth defects are more common among males, and the life expectancy of a boy is a good five years less than that of a newborn girl. One reason for the higher rate of premature death is biological: men lack the oestrogen that protects pre-menopausal women against heart disease. But much of the damage is self-inflicted.

The widest gap in death rates occurs between the ages of 15 and 30 – when men are more than twice as likely as women to die. Accidents, suicide and (to a lesser extent) AIDS are the factors most responsible. Accidental death, frequently associated with drink and driving, reflects what Dr Ian Banks, a Northern Ireland GP, describes as a "James Dean attitude to self-preservation". Risk-taking is a traditional male trait. But the high and rising rate of suicide among young men, which accounts for one in five deaths in this age group, is more difficult to explain.

"Women are better than men at expressing depression and so turn less to suicide," says Dr Banks. "They also have a social network allowing them to discuss their emotions." Denied other avenues of expression, men's negative feelings are more likely to find outlet in aggression, alcohol and drug abuse, and, ultimately, in suicide.

A second bulge in male mortality occurs between the ages of 55 and 70, when a lifetime's smoking shows up as lung cancer, as well as continued high rates of heart disease. But the gender gap in mortality at these ages is likely to narrow over the next decade. The proportion of men smoking has fallen to around 30 per cent, little more than the figure for women. The trend in male lung-cancer deaths is now downward, while that for women is rising steadily. On the other hand, excessive drinking is more than twice as common among men as women.

Male doctors collude with male patients

It is not just risk-taking and hard living that contributes to ill health and early deaths. Men simply resist seeking medical advice. Even when family planning and pregnancy are discounted, women use GP services far more frequently than men. Women consult about prevention; and they consult early with problems. Most men, it is believed, are reluctant to report symptoms that conflict with a self-image of strength and fitness, and have difficulty accepting the loss of control that follows the admission of illness. A recent study from the University of Exeter suggests such ideas are deeply rooted. Among 12-year-olds, twice as many boys as girls say they would not discuss a health problem with anyone.

"Men and women have different perceptions of health," says Peter Williamson, of the East Midlands Men's Health

A foreign correspondent in medicine

Network. "Men tend to perceive their bodies as machines which occasionally need fixing. It is more difficult to take on the sick role, which conflicts with society's stereotype of male behaviour."

These problems are well reflected in the publication *The Crisis in Men's Health*, produced by five men who came together in 1991 to form a men's health awareness project. "We are so detached from our feelings and bodies that we don't notice the danger signals," they write. "Hiding from the messy, physical reality of their lives, many men focus their energy on external goals in the public sphere." Where men do pay attention to their bodies, they do so in a simplistic way. "Working out at the gym, body-building and jogging can become quick-fix activities which have their own dangers," the report argues.

Gay men may have something to teach the wider male world. "Many gay men find it easier to express personal needs and seek help quickly either within their community or from health services. They also have a more effective social support network," says Peter Williamson. This instinct towards openness has been amplified by 15 years' experience of dealing with HIV and AIDS; and the gay community could catalyse change in the health attitudes of male society as a whole.

For the moment, though, seeking help is still seen as unmanly. "I'm here because my wife said I should come," is not an uncommon preface to GP consultations. But, according to Dr Banks, even when a man does manage to get himself to a doctor, his overall health may still be disregarded. Male doctors, he argues, are the worst proponents of men's health.

"If a woman comes into surgery with a sore ear but the conversation turns to cancer, it is normal for the doctor to examine the woman's breasts and to teach her self-examination. If a man comes in with a sore ear, unless he specifically wants you to examine his testicles for signs of cancer, that will not happen," Dr Banks says. "In effect, the male doctor colludes with a male patient in not doing a commonsense check."

GPs are now being encouraged to undertake some forms of routine screening with male patients. "When a woman comes for a smear or advice on contraception, we would routinely measure blood pressure and sugar in the urine," says Dr Andrew Surawy, a GP from Battersea, south London. "But we would now suggest such opportunistic screening with many men."

At last, then, interest in men's health may be moving away from the commercial. The saturation of the women's cosmetics and health market made men an obvious target and three men's health magazines, *Men's Health*, *Maxim* and *XL*, have sprung up in the last year. *Men's Health*, which is upping publication from the current six to 10 issues a year, now has a greater emphasis on genuine health matters, rather than body image.

This interest, coupled with changes in GP attitudes towards health promotion, may do something to tilt men towards better health. But wider social factors are set to thwart improvements. First, evidence suggests that men who live alone (especially the divorced) suffer more ill-health than those who live with a female partner. With rising rates of family break-up, more men than ever are sailing solo through much of their lives.

Second, employment trends are not conducive to better health. While one in 10 men has no job at all, many of those in work do the job of two. "Excessive employment demands promote physical and psychological ill-health and discourage early action to resolve problems," says Dr Surawy, who has noticed increasing levels of stress among his male patients. "With a work culture in which only the fittest survive, no one will admit to weakness."

Meanwhile, in a society which has not yet accepted that breadmaker can be as valid a male role as breadwinner, evidence continues to accumulate showing that lack of a job destroys masculine self-esteem and undermines health. Dr Tony Delamothe, deputy editor of the *British Medical Journal*, has a long-standing interest in poverty and illness. "To the effects of unemployment itself you have to add those of deprivation," he says. "The holes in the safety net are getting bigger. Many men pay the price of increasing social inequality with their health. Some are paying for it with their lives."

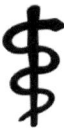

Let's just measure your aorta, sir

The Independent February 1996

Peter Brooker is lucky to be alive. A retired businessman in his mid-sixties, he was last year admitted to hospital for surgery on the bowel. While he was on the operating table, surgeons noticed that his aorta, the main artery that carries

Let's just measure your aorta, sir

blood from the heart to the lower body, was abnormally enlarged. Fit, in fact, to burst. As soon as Mr Brooker recovered from one operation he was back in theatre to have his aorta repaired. He made a good recovery.

George Mason was not so fortunate: he died last year of a ruptured aorta. There were no warning signs and Mr Mason, a publican, also in his sixties, was dead within hours of first becoming ill.

About 5,000 people, three-quarters of them men, die each year following a rupture of the aorta. The death toll from this aortic aneurysm is steadily rising. Most of these deaths could be prevented by screening to detect the abnormal ballooning out of the blood vessel that precedes its bursting. The ultrasound examination needed is quick, safe and simple enough to be carried out in GPs' surgeries.

Yet Gloucestershire is the only health authority in the country to have set up a screening programme for aortic aneurysms. During the past five years, 80 per cent of all men aged 65 and over in the county have had the size of their aortas measured. The normal aorta can be as large in cross-section as a 50p piece. People with aortas double that diameter are advised to have a corrective operation, in which a tube of the artificial fibre dacron is inserted within the weakened section of the blood vessel.

Fifty such operations have been carried out among the 10,000 Gloucestershire men who have been screened so far. The 5 per cent of men whose aortas were larger than normal, but not large enough for immediate surgery, are being followed up in the community or as hospital outpatients.

Controversies over screening for other conditions, such as prostate cancer, show that trying to diagnose disease at a stage before it causes symptoms is not always straightforward. A much-enlarged aorta may still not burst, so screening could lead to unnecessary treatment. And even with the best surgeons, correcting an aortic aneurysm is a tricky procedure. Up to five in 100 patients die as a result of the operation, so early detection has potential drawbacks as well as benefits. "Research is needed to determine the cost-effectiveness of screening," says Dr Maclean Baird, medical spokesman for the British Heart Foundation.

However, those who have put screening into practice take a different view. "If an undiagnosed aneurysm bursts, there is only a 10 per cent chance of survival," says Brian Heather, vascular surgeon at Gloucestershire Royal Hospital. "We are seeing a definite reduction in cases of rupture coming in for emergency surgery. Screening will save lives. The question is one of cost and political acceptability. The lives saved are of relatively elderly men. They may be unproductive in economic terms - but many have a lot to live for."

Postscript

In 2009, the NHS started to offer ultrasound screening for aortic aneurysm to men as they reach 65 years. By 2016, one million men had been screened and 11,000 aneurysms that required treatment or monitoring had been detected.

Chapter Eight

Matters in mind

Whether serious mental illness is linked to creativity is an age-old debate fueled by striking examples such as the poet Sylvia Plath, who suffered from bipolar disorder. But such memorable associations – like rock stars dying at the age of twenty-seven – may mask the far more frequent instances when there is no connection.

It is rare to find an unbiased way of approaching the question. So I was interested to hear of such a study at a psychiatry meeting in 2018 – especially since it related to an article I'd written 25 years earlier in *The Independent*.

AN ICELANDIC SAGA

Iceland is beloved of researchers because it has a small and relatively homogeneous population well disposed towards medical research. In this case, early 90,000 Icelanders took part in a study which calculated their risk of schizophrenia or bipolar disorder based on whether or not they had inherited many hundreds of genes each of which contribute a small increased risk of developing one or both conditions.

Researchers found that having a high overall genetic risk score predicted to a small but significant extent the likelihood that an individual would enter a "creative" career, as defined by membership of the Icelandic national societies of actors, dancers, musicians, visual artists or writers.

They found no such relationship between polygenic risk score for bipolar disorder or schizophrenia and likelihood of employment in other professions such as farming, fishing, manual labour or being an executive.

WRITERS OF INSIGHT AND INSANITY

The Independent March 1993

Gwen Watkins' youngest son, Tristan, suffered for 20 years from manic depression and died two years ago. Her husband, the poet Vernon Watkins, who died in 1967, experienced a severe schizophrenic breakdown when he was a young man.

Vernon Watkins was ill for 18 months. During that period, in addition to completing about 2,000 poems, he slapped the face of a future Archbishop of Canterbury. Tristan was also amazingly productive during his manic phases. "He simply could not type fast enough to get his ideas on to the page," Mrs Watkins recalls.

Mrs Watkins, who lectures on English literature, felt that even a short family history such as hers pointed to two things: that mental instability and creative energy were closely linked; and that a tendency to both could be inherited. She decided to delve more deeply into the apparent connections suggested by the experiences of her husband and son, by carrying out a more general study.

The belief that great imagination involves at least a dash of madness can be traced as far back as the Romans. More recently a study by a geneticist, J L Karlsson, found that a third of the giants of literature experienced episodes of at least borderline insanity, compared with the one-in-20 risk of mental illness in the general population.

But although this indicates a strong association between instability and creativity, it does not explain it. To explore why inspiration and madness should span the generations, Mrs Watkins joined forces with Ruth Pryor, also an authority on English literature, and Dr Gordon Claridge, lecturer in abnormal psychology at Oxford University. Their research has provided new insights into the links between creativity and mental illness, and may modify our attitudes towards the mentally ill.

"Tragic though insanity is, the closeness of the link with creativity signals some hope for those likely to suffer from it," Dr Claridge says. "Since psychosis contains within itself the occasional capacity for superlative functioning and high achievement, we suggest at the very least that those who are mentally ill should not be dismissed as 'merely insane'."

Mrs Watkins has taught English literature from Swansea to Washington, and was a friend of Dylan Thomas. Her book *Sounds from the Bell Jar*, written with Dr Claridge and Ms Pryor explores the links between psychosis and creativity in ten literary figures. But she does not wish to imply that madness is the same as creativity. To paraphrase Sylvia Plath, when you are insane you are too busy being crazy to be anything else.

"Nor would I argue that all creative authors must be mad or carry the propensity to madness," she adds. "There are people like Chaucer and Jane Austen who were inescapably sane, as were their families, as far as we know. However, periods of madness clearly do not preclude great originality of thought. And the overall closeness of association suggests that we might do well to modify our views about the social acceptability of insanity."

Geneticists have investigated the close relatives of psychiatric patients and found that they are more than twice as likely to be authors as the close relatives of a control population. The picture is similar when the association is studied in reverse, by taking a population of writers and looking for psychosis in their families. One such study – of participants in the University of Iowa Writers' Workshop, which spawned such authors as Kurt Vonnegut and Philip Roth – found that the families of the writers were 'riddled' with mental illness as well as creativity.

Families share environments as well as genes. However studies of adoption cases show that both creativity and mental illness follow the line of the natural parents and not that of the adoptive families. What is it that is being inherited? Evidence suggests that it is both a tendency to particular patterns of thought and a set of characteristic emotional responses.

Dr Claridge is struck by the similarities in cognitive style between creative and psychotic thought. These include emphasis on fantasy, divergent thinking and loosely associated ideas. The imagination has been described as having an accelerator but no brake. In a classic American study, psychiatrists were presented with the writings of James Joyce and a number of psychotic patients. Almost half thought that the Joyce excerpts had come from a schizophrenic.

Dr Claridge says: "In schizophrenia, patients cannot limit the contents of consciousness. They are overwhelmed by thoughts which would normally be selected out. One stimulus sets off an uncontrolled series of associations, many bizarre. Creative people are perhaps those who can surrender themselves to that and yet come back."

Studies of the backgrounds of prolific writers such as Virginia Woolf, Sylvia Plath and John Ruskin have revealed threads of madness and creativity running through their family histories. Certain members of the family, it seems, are greatly gifted; others are mad; and many are both. The most likely explanation is that the genes coding for creativity also code for madness, and that the tendency to one is inherited along with the other.

Dr Claridge believes that there is some gateway through which the raw material of creativity must pass from the unconscious to the conscious mind. He suggests that this may be related to anatomical connections between the intuitive right hemisphere of the brain and the language-using, logical left hemisphere.

A resemblance in cognitive style characterises psychotic and imaginative thought. There is also a similarity between the creative and the mad in the intensity of emotional response. Virginia Woolf's father, Leslie Stephen, talked about his 'skinlessness', meaning an almost painful hypersensitivity.

Along with this may go a paradoxical lack of empathy for the feelings of others, perhaps as a means of coping, or perhaps because such people are preoccupied with their own feelings. "This swinging between hypersensitivity and coldness is seen in clinical psychosis," says Dr Claridge.

If inspiration and mental illness are so closely allied, can society do anything to protect those vulnerable individuals endowed with exceptional creativity against the potentially dark side of their gift?

One suggestion is that children who show an unusual degree of imagination might benefit from counselling to enable them to channel their creativity and harden them against clinical psychosis. Another possibility is that ultra-sensitive children might be given help in minimising stress or limiting its effects.

Mrs Watkins also believes that the stigma of mental illness may lead us to underestimate its prevalence in literary figures: "The wild and drunken writer is tolerated, especially if a poet, whereas a psychotic would not be. Dylan Thomas was an alcoholic, but many people use alcohol to mask the symptoms of schizophrenia. He was probably a borderline schizoid personality. And an interpretation of Dylan Thomas's terminal hallucinations as undiagnosed psychosis, rather than as DTs, is now being prepared," she says.

The author John Fowles has talked about writers as those who suffer and go mad for society's sake. Is it of any comfort to Mrs Watkins to think that her son's illness reflects the dark side of a process responsible for creativity?

She has little sympathy for the view that artists exist so that we can stay sane. "What you see is only the extreme suffering. What you see is the waste," she says. "But it seems that people do go mad so that society can have great creative minds. For many, literature is a salvation; for others, a crucifixion."

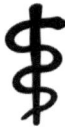

I'M NOT DIOGENES, I JUST COLLECT THINGS

The Independent August 1994

When one of Steve Jones' elderly aunts was forced by disability to move into a residential home, she left him a substantial flat to clear. "Every surface was piled high with rubbish," he says. "It was as if nothing that came into the flat ever left it. You moved from one room to another through corridors of cardboard boxes."

There were spent matches, flat batteries, used tea bags, old tin cans, enough bottles of pills to stock a pharmacy, piles of polystyrene trays, bunches of rusted keys from homes left decades ago, every Christmas and birthday card, copies of the Radio Times going back 17 years, every bill demanded and each receipt for money paid: utilities, public and private, rates, community charge and council tax. There was even one large matchbox full of white cat fur, and one of black.

The phenomenon is not new; the psychologist William James described it in 1890. Moving in to clear a "miser's den" in Boston, public health officials encountered "bushels of such miscellany as is to be found only at the city dump". Such hoarding was, James wrote, a perversion of the natural acquisitive instinct found in everyone.

We all collect something or other, and the value of much of what we collect is arbitrary. Why should stamps be more sought-after than bus tickets? But there is a point when the inability to dispose of worthless objects becomes pathological. It is a phenomenon doctors include in the "Diogenes syndrome". Whether the ancient Greek philosopher ever lived in a barrel is immaterial. His disdain for an ordered household is legendary.

Mr Jones' aunt had the collecting mania and he had the difficult task of sifting through the debris of her life. But in other respects he was lucky. She did not have the complete self-neglect that is the other manifestation of the syndrome. In extreme cases, it can lead to piles of rotting food and even faeces and pools of urine among the assembled junk. That is frequently what leads neighbours or relatives to alert the social and medical services.

Sometimes there is clear mental illness, such as severe depression and dementia, or physical disability. But up to half of all people with Diogenes syndrome appear to be reasonably fit. "Every psychiatrist has two or three such cases on their books," says Dr Mike Nowers, consultant in old age psychiatry at the Cosham Hospital, Bristol. "The question is whether these people too are really ill, or just odd."

It used to be thought that Diogenes syndrome was a personality problem, that these people were just two standard deviations away from the "normal" collector, and that they chose to live in conditions most of us would regard as intolerable. But it has recently been suggested that the syndrome may be due to subtle damage to the frontal lobe of the brain, an area responsible for much of our ability to plan and look after ourselves.

This distinction is not merely academic; it has implications for what can legitimately and ethically be done to help. Under the Mental Health Act of 1983, people can be compulsorily removed to hospital if they are suffering from a mental disorder (which is not defined) and if to do so is in the interest of their own health and safety or for the protection of others. If there is no such mental disorder, a place in a hospital or home can be offered under the National Assistance Act, but it cannot be insisted upon.

The difficulty was recently raised in letters to the *Bulletin of the Royal College of Psychiatrists*. While recognising the severity of the problem, correspondents made clear that they did not wish to act as "agents of social control" who were responsible for "pitchforking elderly people into institutional tidiness". But that situation would change if there was agreed evidence of genuine mental disorder.

Dr Nowers is uncommitted about whether organic brain disease or eccentricity underlies Diogenes syndrome. "It may seem strange to us to sit in squalor, but if that is what people choose to do, what am I to say about it? On the other hand, if you could establish that there is frontal lobe damage then a person's indifference to their state could be seen as part of the problem, and not a true choice. So there is substance behind the debate. Having said that, if I had a pound for every time the frontal lobe had been blamed for some condition or other, I'd be a rich man."

There is now some prospect that the issue will be sorted out. Dr Michael Philpot, consultant in psychogeriatrics at Lewisham and Guy's Mental Health Trust, hopes to start a systematic study of the 200 or so cases of Diogenes Syndrome known to his local social service departments. He aims to conduct a full psychiatric interview with as many as he can. "Hopefully, we will have CT scanning of brain anatomy as part of the study," he says. "We may also be able to use other scanning to show how the frontal lobes are functioning, even if there is no sign that brain structure is abnormal."

Until such research is completed, people with Diogenes syndrome will remain in a diagnostic limbo. Where homes are insanitary, social service "dirty squads" will continue to clean them, only to find conditions deteriorate once the elderly person is back in residence. Poverty seems not to be a contributory factor. A GP in Southampton reported that £15,000 was found among piles of old newspapers in a house lived in by an old lady who chose to dress in rags. So provision of more financial resources is unlikely to make a difference. Other assistance also has little record of success. Even the most hardened home helps give up in despair.

There is a possibility that the hoarding element could be treated using a new class of antidepressants called serotonin reuptake inhibitors. These drugs (of which Prozac is an example) have recently been licensed for use in people with obsessional problems, and collecting mania arguably falls into this category. But Mr Jones' aunt, for one, is unlikely to agree to the need for such treatment.

She argues that she has always been just one step ahead of the recycling movement. The need for her tin cans and newspapers has already been recognised. She confidently expects the time will come for her batteries, polystyrene trays and tea bags. As for the cat fur, the explanation was that it would one day be used to desensitise people with cat allergies. So there *was* a kind of logic.

Mr Jones acknowledges the need for care and sensitivity in sorting through the relics of other people's lives. "Why didn't I junk the lot? Because among all the detritus were things of sentimental value important to family history. My aunt was a gifted diarist and photographer. Some letters and pictures were certainly worth keeping. The least we can expect of those who follow is that they will consider what we have done and conserve anything that may be of value."

Postscript

Dr Philpot's study, published in 2000 in the *Lancet*, found that 70% of people living in extreme squalor had a mental illness. Half of these people had had no contact with mental health services in the previous year. But there were cases not explained by any psychiatric problem or physical disability. The paper does not report the results of brain scans.

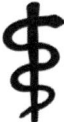

Cognitive behaviour therapy could reasonably be seen as the most significant advance in the past forty years of efforts to help people with mental health problems.

How one man panicked – and survived

The Guardian March 1993

John's problem emerged as he was driving. He was fighting for breath and had a pain in his chest. His feet, hands and mouth were tingling. His vision went black. He was convinced he was having a heart attack and would wake up in intensive care, if at all. Cars were hooting from all sides. He managed to open the window and shout for help, but no one came.

He was actually suffering a severe panic attack: a vicious spiral of fear which turns innocent physical sensations into feelings of imminent catastrophe.

One in 10 of us has a similar experience at some stage. Although exhaustive physical examination showed John to be fit, the attacks worsened. He had to give up his job as a BBC radio producer. A five-mile car journey could take two hours. He crashed twice in a year.

Every time he went out he thought the symptoms would recur – and they did. "I saw it as a malevolent external force – a demon come to get me. It found a way into my house, so that I wasn't safe even there. I felt I'd die and no one would know. So I used to sit on the wall outside or walk up and down the road. And no one could comfort me by giving it a name."

However, help was at hand: clinical psychologist Dr David Clark was developing a new treatment at the Warneford Hospital, Oxford. John saw him for three months. "Within six weeks I was driving the car again, and working. Not only was the immediate problem cleared up, but I recognised that feelings of near panic had been part of my life for many years."

John has a natural tendency to over-breathe, or hyperventilate, when anxious. This puts excess oxygen into the bloodstream, blows off carbon dioxide and causes "tingling". The sensations are normal, though if you perceive them as alarming, they will be.

"Once you start you're trapped in a spiral", says John. "You hyperventilate more and the symptoms worsen. But once you know the explanation, the sensations cease to be worrying. It's a dandelion clock of an affliction. One blow from the right quarter and it ceases to exist".

The road to Damascus experience came when Clark and he did some over-breathing together. Two middle aged men sitting there huffing and puffing. "All the sensations recurred. Then David said in a commanding voice 'Stand up'. And I did, and I didn't faint. All my fears were refuted in one go. I remember laughing with a genuinely light heart."

John, who's now driving again, had "cognitive therapy". Treatment starts with careful questioning about the events before an attack and the thoughts accompanying it. Discussion and experiment help to explain worrying bodily sensations (excessive heart rate, difficult breathing, dizziness and a sense of unreality). Clinical trials show therapy works in about 90 per cent of cases and is better than commonly prescribed drugs and relaxation training.

Over-breathing is not the only cause of panic attacks. Sufferers share a tendency to scan their bodies repeatedly for signs of danger. This hypervigilance alerts them to a whole variety of sensations other people may be unaware of. Such sensations can be misinterpreted as evidence of a serious physical disorder, encouraging catastrophic beliefs, at great cost to lifestyle. For example, those who see occasional palpitations as evidence of a weak heart may stop exercise in the belief that it will prevent a fatal attack.

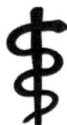

ACCENTUATE THE POSITIVE

The Independent May 1989

Optimists have fewer illnesses and more successful careers.

Half the five thousand salesmen recruited by a US insurance company quit within a year, unable to stand the rejection from nine of every ten people they approached. A life so rich in disappointment is a good testbed for ideas about what makes certain people psychologically resilient.

So Martin Seligman, of the University of Pennsylvania, used insurance salesmen to test his theory that a fundamental optimism – a feature he describes as having a "Yes" in your heart – underpins achievement and psychological health.

Professor Seligman gave a questionnaire to fifteen thousand applicants who sat the standard professional qualification for life insurance salesmen. One thousand were hired. From their responses, roughly half were optimists, half pessimists.

The company also took on a special force of 129 people who failed the exam but were particularly optimistic by the questionnaire. Over the next two years, the optimists in the regular workforce significantly outsold the pessimists, but the special force of super-optimists outperformed everyone. The optimism measure promises to cut training costs and relieve the misery of those unsuited to the job. It may also help in selecting athletes.

At the University of Berkeley, the Seligman questionnaire has been given to top class swimmers. Results seem to predict both the number of sub-standard performances in a season (pessimists have more) and how swimmers respond to a disappointing performance: optimists better their time when sent back into the pool while pessimists do still worse.

Perhaps most remarkable of all, the theory fits the outcome of US presidential elections. By analysing nomination speeches, Martin Seligman and colleagues have assessed the explanatory style of every candidate since 1900. In 18 of the last 23 contests, the candidate with the more optimistic explanatory style has reached the White House.

Such predictive power is rare in psychological theories. Can the way we make sense of what happens to us really be scientifically investigated?

When something bad happens, people naturally ask why. The causes they come up with can be classified along three dimensions. The first is internal/external: was the disaster due to me, or to other people or circumstances? Then there is the *stability* of the cause. Did it apply only then, or will it be true forever? This is the difference between "he's rotten" and "all men are rotten" when explaining the breakup of a relationship. Finally, there is the question of whether the cause is specific or global: does it apply just to this kind of event, or to everything?

A standard example is how people might react to exam failure. "It's my fault. I always fail exams. I guess it's because I'm stupid" is a pessimistic explanation: internal, stable and global. "I failed because the exam was hard. This time things didn't work out. And, anyway, I'm worse at maths than other subjects" is the answer of an optimist.

Pessimists are much more likely to become depressed. "This explanatory style is a risk factor for depression just as cigarette smoking is a risk factor for lung cancer," Dr

Seligman says. One striking study shows that the lasting effects of therapy depend very much on altering the way depressed people construe events. Patients were treated with antidepressant drugs or received therapy. At the end of treatment, which was successful in most cases, explanatory style was assessed.

Some patients had become optimistic, while others remained pessimists – even though their depressive symptoms had improved to much the same extent. Over the next two years, the pessimists showed a far greater tendency than the optimists to relapse into depression.

Several studies indicated that pessimists also have poorer physical health. A strong source of evidence is from a cohort of Harvard students. Open-ended questionnaire responses from an early phase of the study have been scored for optimism/pessimism. From middle age onwards, the pessimists become substantially more prone than optimists to chronic diseases of ageing.

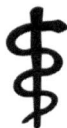

ELIMINATE THE NEGATIVE

Medical Monitor March 1992

Cognitive therapists tell a story that illustrates how the same situation can evoke different emotional responses in different people, depending on habitual patterns of thought.

Eliminate the negative

Four men leave for work one morning. Each steps straight onto a dog turd. The first thinks: "Oh shit, I can't even get down the drive without messing things up. I'm a complete failure. I might as well go back to bed." This is the person inclined to depression.

The second thinks: "Oh shit, I'll never clean this up in time for my train. Then I'll lose my job and my wife will leave me." This is the anxious person.

The third man, who suffers from excessive anger, thinks: "It's that bastard with the alsatian at number 76. I'll knock his fucking head off."

The fourth, who has had cognitive therapy, thinks: "Oh shit. But thank goodness I'm wearing shoes today."

Cognitive therapy was developed in Philadelphia by the psychiatrist Aaron Beck, who argued that negative thinking is not so much a symptom of depression as a cause of it. The aim of therapy is to eliminate negative thoughts by challenging patients' beliefs and assumptions in a process of guided discovery in which patient and therapist collaborate.

The first phase is to identify a patient's specific problems. Once specific difficulties are distinguished from the morass, they may seem more manageable. The second stage is to systematically explore the assumptions that a patient holds about the world. These assumptions may have arisen in childhood, but can also be the result of more recent experience. People are often unaware that they hold fixed "rules about life" that can colour their every experience.

One assumption characteristic of depressed patients is that they must be successful to be worthwhile. This has the merit of motivating much positive activity but can be counterproductive if held in an extreme form that makes patients susceptible to the effects of failure, even of relatively minor kinds. A feature of depression is that cognitive distortions are entrenched. Patients attend selectively to events which reinforce negative beliefs, interpreting experiences as evidence of defeat and inadequacy. They may also engage in self defeating behaviours which confirm these views.

In a case such as that of a woman with depression who felt unable to cope with the demands of a job and housework, the dysfunctional assumption might be that she has to be completely competent to avoid being a failure. The therapist might say "Do you know anyone who is 100% perfect? What is the worst thing that could happen if you don't wash up? What would be the family's reaction if the ironing was late? Would it really be that bad? Maybe you could get one of them to help with it."

It may be that part of the problem was early experience of a highly competent mother who punished the woman if she failed to do enough or pleased herself rather than others. But, unlike dynamic psychotherapy such as Freudian analysis, such childhood experience would be explored only if relevant to current problems.

Another difference is that cognitive therapists from the outset have tried to evaluate their success and failure, and refine their techniques, based on the outcome of controlled clinical trials.

Chapter Nine

Not all brilliant ideas have a bright future

FINDING THE WAY HOME

World Medicine February 1981

Do we have a magnetic sense?

If you treat human beings like homing pigeons, they behave like them – or so say zoologists at Manchester University who have demonstrated a magnetic sense of direction in man. People totally confused about the route that have been taken *can* accurately point the way home. Dr Robin Baker and his colleagues also claim to have located the internal compass, under the olfactory lobes of the brain.

For the past two years, coachloads of blindfolded students have been traversing northwest England on tortuous journeys. When they arrive at their unknown destinations they are asked to point to the place they've come from. Although convinced they are guessing wildly, subjects show a surprising degree of accuracy. There is good agreement in their judgments and the average direction indicated is usually very close to the true compass bearing. Robin Baker thought at first that people might be using the direction of the sun as a clue. Together with the (extremely sceptical) "props" department of Yorkshire Television he arranged an experiment to refute this idea.

A foreign correspondent in medicine

A group of sixth-form children was divided into two. One half carried brass bars on the back of their heads, tucked into the elastic of their blindfolds; the other carried bar magnets. The children with the brass bars judged the direction correctly; those with magnets didn't. This seemed fairly convincing, so Robin Baker then carried out a series of more sophisticated experiments.

In these, the direction of the magnetic lines of force through the head were systematically varied using battery-powered helmets. On the basis of these experiments, the Manchester team has predicted that the internal compass will be found under the olfactory lobes. Although still to be confirmed by histology and by magnetometer tests, the proposed site looks reasonable, for in wood-mice small permanent magnets (probably magnetite) have already been found in tissue taken from that area of the brain.

Of course we have known of a directional sense in animals for many years. At appropriate seasons, caged migratory birds hop in the direction they should be travelling, while the navigational feats of bees, cats, and pigeons are legendary. But why should man have the same abilities? Dr Baker suggests the advantage lies simply in being able more effectively to explore unknown territory. Remembering a series of changes in direction is inefficient, and navigating by landmarks unreliable; what better way of solving the problem than one's very own built-in set of compass needles?

Postscript

Attempts in the USA to replicate Robin Baker's Manchester experiments failed, but there has continued to be some interest in the possibility that humans have a magnetic sense. In 2019 Joseph Kirschvink, of the California Institute of Technology, claimed to have evidence that electrical activity in the human brain can be influenced by changes in magnetic field. But no-one has located a site in the brain containing any internal compass (if such a thing exists).

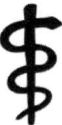

Is there anything there?

World Medicine May 1982

Cambridge parapsychologist Carl Sargent claims to have sound experimental evidence for the existence of extrasensory perception.

That a Californian university should boast it own professor of parapsychology is not difficult to believe, but for Cambridge University to be seriously investigating the paranormal is somewhat unlikely. That the experiments should produce convincing evidence for the reality of extrasensory perception is less likely still. But this is what post-doctoral researcher Carl Sargent has come up with after five years of work in the university department of experimental psychology.

His findings should have caused a stir in conventional circles, but have been met with polite disbelief, and their implications largely ignored. Perhaps understandably, Carl

A foreign correspondent in medicine

Sargent is sharply critical of the attitudes of his colleagues and describes much of their work as trivial and boring.

When I went along to be a subject in a parapsychology experiment, I underwent an experience that was bizarre and at times disturbing. Though not wholly convinced, I did at least emerge more inclined to question my scepticism.

The standard ESP experiment involves depriving the ordinary senses. An assistant sellotaped half ping-pong balls over my eyes and played continuous white noise (like the sound of frying fish) to both ears. The only illumination came from a red 60 watt bulb. Functionally blind and deaf, I lay on the floor of a large room. The assistant observed me through a one-way mirror. I then had to describe the images, ideas, and feelings I experienced.

Meanwhile, Carl Sargent, in another building, had four pictures selected at random from pool of 200: a Brueghel landscape, a painting of the Clifton suspension bridge, a "science fiction" illustration, and a child's drawing of two elephants having a bath. Of these the Brueghel was chosen as the target he was to concentrate on "sending". At the end of the session I had to rank the four pictures according to the likelihood they had been the target. I also had to "mark" each picture according to how it matched each image and impression recorded in my transcript.

Not to my surprise, my choice of target was incorrect. But, my performance as a psychic was redeemed by the fact I ranked the true target second; and by the "marks" I had assigned, it proved to have been very close.

Extrasensory perception apart, I was impressed by the bizarre effects of the sensory deprivation itself. The aim of the procedure, known as the Ganzfeld (from the German: whole field) is to reduce any distraction by external events, and it also helps avoid suspicion that the sender might be communicating with the subject through the usual sensory channels. For the same reason, the sender goes not just to another room, but to another building. Carl Sargent admits this may not be absolutely necessary, but it does impress sceptics who think that information is conveyed by banging on the waterpipes.

After the experiment I was asked to judge how long the session had lasted. I thought it might have been fifteen minutes, but estimated ten; in fact my period of sensory deprivation had lasted thirty-five minutes. The time distortion had not been unpleasant but the illusion of movement had. I had a strong feeling that the mattress was being rocked and that I was sharing it with someone else, though I am assured I was not.

What does such an experiment reveal of ESP? Most people believe or disbelieve in the paranormal according to their personal experiences. Illogical it may be, but it does mean that Carl Sargent finds it very difficult to convince sceptics with statistical arguments.

The crucial part of his experiment is whether the picture the subject chooses was the one he transmitted. With four possibilities, the probability of a chance "hit" is 25 per cent for each occasion. Success (or failure) on each individual attempt is therefore less important that the overall rate obtained by large numbers of subjects. So far, Carl Sargent has found an overall success rate of 40 (rather than 25) per cent. This is significantly and repeatedly greater than chance.

Such evidence is impressive enough, but even more disturbing is Sargent's suggestion that the receiver can correctly choose the picture *before* it is selected. So far he has tried only one experiment of this kind. But on eighteen out of forty-four occasions (compared with an expected eleven) the picture eventually selected at random from the four possibles corresponded to one selected earlier by the subject. Such a result would be expected by chance fewer than one time in fifty. Nevertheless, Sargent is cautious about these results, regarding them merely as evidence that there is "something" worth further investigation. He is similarly cautious about labelling the effect. It could be precognition, or it could be psychokinesis, in which the initial choice actually biases any subsequent "random" selection of the target.

I heard Sargent present his findings to a meeting of the MRC Applied Psychology Unit in Cambridge. Psychologists there are a hard-headed bunch, not averse to drawing and quartering visiting speakers. But his reception was subdued: they apparently found little to criticise in his experimental method or statistical interpretation.

As believers in empirical science, we must either accept that the data show ESP really exists, or we must deny the personal integrity of the researcher. Carl Sargent argues that we would be justified in disbelieving his results if they were unique. But he claims that nine independent laboratories in the UK and the USA have produced similar results, and to argue that all these researchers are dishonest would mean postulating an improbably large conspiracy. On a personal level, why *should* he fabricate the data? He came into the field with an open mind, and if he had come out with convincingly *negative* results he would probably be in a much better position within mainstream psychology than he is now.

Carl Sargent thinks the crucial factor is the number of replication laboratories. Turning the tables on his detractors, he asks how many findings in conventional psychology have been replicated nine times: "Very few experiments are ever repeated, because they're so trivial and boring that nobody bothers." This leaves plenty of opportunity for abuse. He argues that social scientists imagine parapsychologists fudge the data because they know such behaviour is not uncommon among their associates. Basically, he says, "Psychologists think we cheat because *they* do." With Sir Cyril Burt in the broom cupboard, it's not easy to deny.

Parapsychology used to consist of a lot of facts but no theory. Now, argues Sargent, it is effectively underpinned, if not exactly by a theory, then at least by a good working metaphor: that ESP behaves like a weak sensory system, in which a signal is detected against a background of "noise". This helps explain why the receiver scores not only a greater than chance number of direct hits, but also a greater than chance number of second choice "near misses".

The analogy of a weak sensory system may give us the feeling that ESP is not so improbable after all. But what of precognition and/or psychokinesis? Sargent argues that radical modern physics not only allows that such phenomena may occur but even insists that they *must* exist. A fairly conventional definition of ESP talks in terms of a "statistically discernible correlation between a response and a stimulus when there is a perfect sensory shielding between the two and when the information is non-inferential".

A more all-encompassing (and Californian) viewpoint asserts that the paranormal is "a breakdown in the laws of probability in the presence of a motivated observer". Sargent argues: "The flavour underlying that is the flavour of quantum physics." In a universe where all laws governing the behaviour of the system are created by the act of observation itself, we would expect the unexpected.

> The most striking example of ESP which has emerged from the Cambridge work concerns Blake's painting *Ancient of Days*. The "receiver" did not know this was one of the 200 pictures, photographs, and cartoons which make up the pool of items from which the one to be "sent" is ultimately drawn. During a sixteen minute session, the receiver reported these images from his stream of consciousness:
>
> *At 3 min 10 secs*: "A picture of a night sky with a planet or some unnatural golden, oval, glowing object with fire coming off it."
>
> *At 6 min 38 secs*: "A figure 8, protracted to infinity, very smooth, getting wider as it comes nearer."
>
> *At 5 min 08 secs*: "Clumsily drawn picture of a woman in white nightdress, ragged hair, torch in one hand, hands and feet too large."
>
> *After 11 min 57 secs*: "Close-up picture of the sun; can see red flames on the surface, the sun looks black."
>
> *At 12 min 25 secs*: "Blake's picture of God with the dividers creating the world."

Postscript

When Carl Sargent died in 2018, an obituary praised his incredible gift for storytelling and the making of myths. This related to his work as a prolific author of fantasy role-playing games such as *Dungeons and Dragons* and *Warhammer*. But there are some who might suggest it could apply equally to his earlier career as a parapsychologist.

In 1979, a fellow parapsychologist spent several days observing Sargent's experiments and concluded that failure to follow procedures scrupulously enough created opportunity for errors or conscious or unconscious bias to influence the results of the ESP experiments.

In 1982, Carl Sargent co-wrote *Explaining the unexplained: mysteries of the paranormal* with Hans Eysenck (of whom, more below).

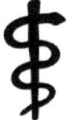

STRING THEORY

World Medicine May 1982

The York meeting of British psychologists heard that intelligence could be measured with a piece of string. Would the idea unravel?

"What's new in the measurement of intelligence?" asked Professor Hans Eysenck in the title of his guest lecture. Part of the answer was that you could measure it very nicely using an EEG trace and a piece of string (though if you didn't have a piece of string, a computer would do the job just as well).

The professor is used to controversy, and some have argued his desire to excite it is the only consistent theme in his distinguished career. The egalitarian establishment was apoplectic at his conclusion that IQ was distributed in less than equal proportions between the races; the medical profession just as outraged at his assertion that smoking was not a proven cause of cancer.

When he suggested that career choice and attainment were subject to astrological influence, he invited understandable incredulity. But how was one to react to this latest novelty in intelligence testing? Was the appropriate critique to be on ideological, methodological or plainly psychiatric grounds?

Eysenck's defenders say that he is a radical empiricist – that he believes what the data tell him, however unlikely or unpopular. This is really an implicit criticism of other scientists who are thought to file uncomfortable results in the back of a bottom draw marked "pending further analysis".

But, unfortunately, Eysenck's ear for what the data say is suspect. What they whisper to him is often different from what they shout at everyone else – *vide* Richard Peto's demolition job on Eysenck's interpretation of the lung cancer statistics.

EEG pattern

But what of the argument in this case? The idea is that the pattern of EEG response produced by brief auditory or visual stimulation varies according to the accuracy with which neural impulses are propagated through the cortex. Where errors in transmission are few, the trace is complex; where they are frequent, the averaged evoked response is smoothed out. So those with an alpine evoked potential are intelligent; those with gentle undulations dull.

The claimed correlation between string or computer-calculated complexity and paper-and-pencil IQ is extremely high. But this may merely reflect limited or lucky sampling of subjects. It may also be due to selecting too many subjects from the extremes of the intelligence dimension, as has been the case with similar associations in the past.

Gentle seething

The reaction of Eysenck's fellow psychologists was difficult to judge since with guest lecturer status no questions were taken or discussion allowed. But a gentle seething and exchange of scribbled bits of paper had been detectable.

Perhaps most telling was the comment that if anyone but Eysenck had presented such results, people would have been interested. But maybe Eysenck isn't concerned any more about exciting the interest of psychologists – even though their threshold for interest is obviously set low. They did, for example, also hear a paper entitled: "A retrospective idealisation of stages along the road towards pragmatic pluralism in psychology". And then there was the other classic contribution to the final day's proceedings: "Counter-attitudinal advocacy-induced self-persuasion and the anticipated consumption of caterpillars." I was assured that title was no joke, though with conferences which begin on April 1 one can never be sure.

Postscript

It was also on 1st April 1982 that the first Argentinian troops landed on the Falkland Islands.

The idea that the complexity of an EEG trace relates to intelligence has not gone away entirely, though those who pursue it now suggest the link is modulated by attentional factors that vary with the task used to elicit the EEG response. Hans Eysenck's reputation, however, has taken a real knock: in 2019, an enquiry by King's College, London, called for many of his papers to be retracted since the size of the effects they reported were inconceivably large.

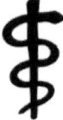

Boosting the output of a failing heart by persuading ordinary muscle to emulate its cardiac equivalent seemed a serious possibility in the 1980s. The idea was that skeletal muscle could be conditioned – by repeated electrical stimulation – to develop a tireless ability to contract, and could then be used to contribute pumping power.

The idea of literally adding muscle to the heart has not, at least not yet, born fruit. But the concept had much going for it. The tissue involved was the patient's own, so there was no need (as with heart transplants) to control rejection; and there is no chronic shortage of donors. Also, mechanical devices to assist the heart were at the time clumsy and cumbersome and beset by problems of power supply.

BACKING UP THE HEART

The Guardian November 1986

Within five years, an auxiliary heart made of ordinary back muscle could be in routine use to boost circulation in patients with heart failure.

Backing up the heart

Heart muscle is rightly regarded as unique, notably in its resistance to fatigue. No other muscle contracts every second or so, day in and day out, for a lifetime. But a new conditioning process, involving repeated electrical stimulation, seems capable of modifying other muscles so that they develop the tirelessness that characterises the heart.

In a joint British and American venture, scientists in Birmingham have joined with surgeons in Philadelphia to explore the potential of the new technique. "Skeletal muscle is highly specialised, but – as we know from the effects of exercise – still capable of adaptation," says Dr Stanley Salmons, from Birmingham University's Department of Anatomy. "I showed that continuous electrical stimulation produces effects of the same type as exercise, but very much greater in extent".

There is increased blood supply, a change in the enzymes that regulate the muscle cells' energy reserves, and a switch from highly fatiguable 'fast' muscle fibres to their more resilient slow-fibre counterparts. The genetic characteristics of the cells – which have the potential to develop into either form of fibre – become re-expressed."

Modifying muscle is stage one. Next comes making it pump. But that is relatively straightforward plastic surgery and a little ingenuity with wires and boxes.

The tissue most likely to be used is the *latissimus dorsi*, the muscle that gives the wedge shape at the back of the armpit. Taking out a portion of the second rib allows the whole of it to be shifted into the chest with all its nerve and blood supply intact. Once there, the muscle is wrapped into a spiral pouch and plumbed into the aorta – the major vessel that takes blood from the heart.

Since the muscle's nerve connections are preserved, the whole artificial chamber, or ventricle, can be stimulated to contract by a simple placement of electrodes attached to one of the new generation of "intelligent" pacemakers that senses the electrical activity of the heart before it acts. The muscle pouch is made to contract as the heart relaxes, giving blood that all-important extra push along the aorta. The body's vital organs are once more effectively supplied with oxygen and nutrients, and the spiral of decline caused by heart failure is reversed.

Research in dogs shows that the auxiliary skeletal muscle pump can do about half the work of the heart's left ventricle – the one that circulates blood to the body – for as long as nine weeks. Stanley Salmons and his surgical colleague Larry Stephenson at the University of Pennsylvania are confident their techniques will soon be applied in patients.

Skeletal muscle is the most efficient means known to man of converting electrical to mechanical energy. And there is plenty of it around that is doing a good job of holding our bones together but which could be put to other use if needed.

Postscript

The idea has never been tried in patients, but Stanley Salmons and colleagues continue to argue that cardiomyoplasty, as the technique is called, is not a failed approach. What we need, they suggest, is a better understanding of how to make the muscle graft more viable and powerful by conditioning it in the clinical context. Given the shortage of heart donors, we urgently need alternatives to transplantation, and this suggestion is still worth pursuing.

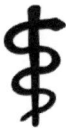

Spurt in Artificial Blood

The Guardian October 1986

Refrigeration fluid may be better than the red stuff.

Imagine a substance that can carry twice as much oxygen as blood, and deliver it up to our tissues twice as fast; that flows into oxygen-deprived parts of the body which blood cannot reach; that can be stored with a shelf-life of years; that can be used without cross-matching donor and patient; and that carries no risk of infection – it is a specification (a haematologist's Heineken and more) that sounds impossible to fulfil.

Yet such liquids exist. They are fluorocarbons: molecules in which hydrogen atoms have been replaced by fluorine. Fluorocarbons are inert and twice as heavy as water. Industry uses them as refrigeration fluids and aerosol propellants. But their fascination for medicine lies in the fact that, in pure form, fluorocarbons dissolve 40–50 litres of oxygen for every 100 litres of fluid.

There are drawbacks of course. But fear of AIDS transmission, plus increasing difficulties in obtaining supplies of transfusable blood, have given new impetus to research aimed at overcoming them. One method – forming artificial blood "cells" by encapsulating fluorocarbons in envelopes made of fats or complex sugars – shows promise.

Dramatic demonstration of the properties of fluorocarbons came in 1966 when Leland Clark in Birmingham, Alabama, submerged a mouse in an oxygenated solution and found it could survive six hours breathing liquid instead of air. But the barrier to widespread use of fluorocarbons is that they do not mix with water. Before we can think of them as an alternative to transfusing blood, we must first turn fluorocarbons into an emulsion using a form of detergent. This seems to introduce adverse effects.

Even so, clinical testing of fluorocarbon "blood" started in 1979, pioneered by the Green Cross Corporation of Osaka and physicians in Japan. A paper in *Annals of Surgery* in 1982 reported that 186 patients had been treated with no untoward reactions.

But this was not so the first time fluorocarbons were used in the US, on an anaemic Jehovah's Witness who had severe haemorrhage after surgery. And the frequency of side effects in subsequent cases made American investigators doubt the honesty of previous claims.

Side effects are thought to arise from the emulsifying agents. These activate proteins in the blood that lead to the clumping of platelets which damage the lungs. So there is great interest in new techniques based on the encapsulation of fluorocarbons. Speaking this summer [1986] at the conference of the European Society of Cardiothoracic Anaesthetists, Dr Patrick Salt, senior lecturer in anaesthesia at Birmingham University, said: "We're now trying to get by without an emulsion. We might have to increase particle size but we could compensate by making the particles more flexible than a red blood cell."

This is an important consideration since fluorocarbon-based

blood substitutes flow more easily than the real thing. Because its droplet size is one seventieth the diameter of a red blood cell, fluorocarbon passes through tiny or partially blocked vessels in which ordinary blood slows and starts to sludge.

Earlier this year in Brussels, a meeting on intensive care and emergency medicine heard evidence that the size of heart attacks in dogs can be reduced by infusing fluorocarbons into the affected area of heart muscle. Simon Faithfull, from Rotterdam's Erasmus University, also claimed that human limbs severed in accidents could be kept viable for up to 72 hours and then successfully reattached if they had been stored in fluorocarbons. Organs awaiting transplantation could be similarly preserved.

Postscript

In January 1991, consultant cardiologist Dr Jonathan Pitts Crick used the fluorocarbon Fluosol in a patient having a coronary artery procedure (balloon angioplasty) at the Bristol Royal Infirmary. This was the first time the blood substitute had been used in the UK. The patient recovered well. In the previous year, the *American Journal of Cardiology* had published a randomised trial comparing Fluosol-assisted balloon angioplasty against the conventional procedure. It looked as if the new technique helped maintain oxygen supply to the heart. But over the following thirty years no fluorocarbon-based artificial blood products have been successfully introduced into clinical practice.

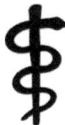

Parkinsonism's "great leap forward"

Pharmacy Update October 1986

The intriguing link between synthetic narcotics and Parkinson's disease is strengthened by recent data discussed at the Royal Institution.

California's contribution to understanding parkinsonism began with a chance meeting between a lawyer and a physicist in Stanford Library. Discussion turned to the design and manufacture of synthetic narcotics that acted like heroin, but were novel enough compounds to escape current legal controls. Their original idea was to write a book on clandestine chemistry; but the two men eventually decided to make drugs instead.

The fruits of their labour first came to clinical attention in the summer of 1982 when a 42-year-old intravenous drug abuser developed a sudden parkinsonian state. He had gone to sleep with his arm round his girlfriend and in the morning was unable to move it, or anything else. He was mute, rigid, drooling and had profound slowness of movement. Suspicion fell on possible impurities in the synthetic drug he had been using. This was confirmed when a public announcement that there was "bad heroin on the street" brought another six cases of Parkinson's syndrome, with intravenous drug use as their only link.

Samples from police raids revealed a compound which fitted none of the 40,000 substances on file. Later investigation showed it to be MPTP, a substance similar to the pethidine

Parkinsonism's "great leap forward"

analogue MPPP, for which the two Californian chemists had been aiming.

Injection of MPTP into primates produced symptoms that were also strikingly like parkinsonism. The condition was reversible by L-dopa; and post-mortem examination showed selective lesions in the dopamine neurones of the substantia nigra in the brain.

These were dramatic events, since there had never been an animal model of the disease, and one was desperately needed for research into its more effective treatment. A century-and-a-half since James Parkinson's original treatise had brought little understanding of the disease. Now there was an agent which, given systemically, homed in on exactly that part of the brain known to be affected in humans, producing what appeared to be a remarkably "pure" parkinsonian state.

But how pure was it? Doubters surfaced quickly. Was the tremor truly parkinsonian? Why were the effects of MPTP confined to the substantia nigra, when real Parkinson's disease was known to produce degeneration in other areas as well? And where were the round, intracellular features called Lewy bodies which so characterise the disease in man?

Speaking at the Royal Institution in April, Bill Langston, the neurologist who first saw the "frozen" addicts of California (and effectively established the MPTP connection) was able to put one doubt to rest.

In four out of seven patients, the tremor occurs at rest, and is very similar to that of Parkinson's disease. Importantly, resting tremor has now also been reproduced in MPTP-injected monkeys.

Other doubts have been answered by looking at the interaction between MPTP effects and age. In monkeys that are middle-aged or older (rather than the usual, young specimens employed for research), Bill Langston and colleagues have now found "unequivocal evidence" of damage, including loss of neurones, spreading beyond the substantia nigra. Crucially, they have also found structures which — if they are not Lewy bodies — are amazingly like them.

"This is the crux," said Professor David Marsden, of the Institute of Psychiatry. "If you've produced something that is very nearly a Lewy body, you've produced something that is very nearly Parkinson's disease."

The outcome of the debate is far from academic. Throughout the world, many thousands of sufferers from parkinsonism are hoping that MPTP truly is the key to the control of the disease. There are also at least 400 people from California's drug-taking fraternity anxious that researchers come up with an answer.

The MPTP story has far to run. Already it is full of characters, and irony. There is, for example, the clandestine chemist responsible for the Californian MPTP epidemic who told the police his experiments were aimed at creating a new hand lotion; and who persevered with them despite a fire that sent his clandestine laboratory up in flames and scattered like confetti the papers on psychotropic drug synthesis that he had carefully razored from journals in the Stanford library. He is now in jail with what looks like a developing parkinsonian syndrome.

But the biggest irony of all is that the therapeutic potential of MPTP was actively research by drug companies in the 1950s, until deaths among volunteers led to the abandonment of all trials. The disease they thought it might cure was parkinsonism.

Postscript

The MPTP model proved a useful research tool. But the events surrounding MPTP did not bring the long hoped-for identification of an environmental toxin responsible for Parkinson's Disease. We are still wrestling with a degenerative disorder of complex pathology, uncertain cause (though gene mutations are involved in some people) and relatively short-lived response to therapy.

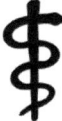

Bone marrow banking "could soothe nuclear fears"

Hospital Doctor March 1987

Bone marrow may one day be harvested commercially and stored in the deep-freeze, the Rome Symposium on Acute Leukaemias was told. Transplant of the harvested marrow could benefit donors who develop leukaemia or lymphoma. And it is suggested that workers in the nuclear power industry would feel happier for having marrow stored in case of Chernobyl-style disaster.

The idea of private bone marrow banks emerged at the UICC cancer congress last year in Budapest. Around 700ml of marrow is taken from the pelvis. Removal of the red cells leaves concentrated stem cells which then have a preservative added and are frozen, maintaining their ability to reconstitute the immune system.

Having marrow in storage in case of blood cancers is one thing, since we control the dose of radiation used to destroy the malignant marrow which needs replacement. The situation following uncontrolled radiation exposure is quite different, as Robert Gale found after Chernobyl, when the only way radiation dose could be judged was by seeing how fast the patient's white cell count fell.

Those closest to the radiation source die of neurological damage almost immediately. Those a little further away suffer gastrointestinal death after a few days. Bone marrow response is relevant only in people receiving a relatively small dose, perhaps 200–800 rads, and even that is critically dependent on rate of exposure. So only a small proportion of those affected stand any chance of salvage.

Even so, having a large freezer well away from Whitehall or Sellafield sounds like an attractive proposition for key politicians, administrators and the military as a precaution against nuclear war. Doctors approached have been keen to point out that they too would need to survive to supervise marrow transplantation.

As for routine commercial harvesting, those floating the idea suggest a mere 5ml would contain enough stem cells for the marrow to be reconstituted. There was evidence at the Rome meeting that stem cells harvested from peripheral blood could also do the job, which would really put commercial marrow preservation on the map.

Postscript

Generally, we do now harvest blood-forming stem cells from circulating blood and not from marrow extracted from the bones. Robert Gale, a radiation expert at the University of California

Bone marrow banking "could soothe nuclear fears"

Los Angeles, travelled to the then Soviet Union at the invitation of Mikhail Gorbachev to help with the treatment of survivors of the 1986 Chernobyl nuclear accident. It is not clear whether bone marrow transplantation saved any lives. Since then, harvesting bone marrow has not become a viable commercial proposition.

Chapter Ten

Cancer: playing the long game

Over decades of talking to US doctors, I've noticed that remarkably few of them "get" the NHS. The US system is highly effective at world class care for those who can afford it, but this is achieved at great financial cost and still greater cost in social equality. There are undoubted inefficiencies in the NHS, but there are also remarkable perverse incentives in the profit-driven model of US healthcare.

I witnessed one striking example in the 1990s at an advisory board of US cancer specialists held in Florida for a UK pharma company[1]. The company was outlining how their research was likely to replace many complex intravenous cancer treatments with a once-daily pill that was targeted precisely at tumour cells, far more convenient for patients, and had fewer side effects. Wouldn't this be a great thing all-round?

One US doctor agreed. He worked for the Veterans' Administration, which provides healthcare for ex-military personnel and is the closest the US comes to the NHS ideal. The others looked very sceptical. The reason was that much of their income came from

---

[1] Another experience is relevant. I was arranging interviews with US and UK specialists to sound out their interest in helping with clinical trials. One US doctor said he would agree to my visit only if we paid him twice the several hundred dollars we initially offered. In contrast, a UK doctor said he did not want any payment for himself but would like us to make a contribution to Mountain Rescue. That said, he continued, I have to declare an interest: "I would like it to be the Lake District mountain rescue, since this is the service I am most likely to need."

giving intravenous cancer drugs, and very little would be forthcoming from prescribing a pill. So this was a prospect that left them feeling rather nauseous. "Smart" drugs have come, nevertheless.

The need for targeted drugs

In a cell that gives rise to cancer, several abnormal things happen. First, and most obviously, the cell starts to reproduce itself far more frequently than is required for the repair and replacement of tissue. Secondly, it loses its ability to self-destruct: generally, severely abnormal cells die, but cells that have undergone malignant transformation find ways of bypassing our bodies' protective mechanism.

Thirdly, when cancer cells group together, they begin to secrete molecules that cause neighbouring healthy cells to form blood vessels that bring the tumour the oxygen and nutrients it needs for rapid growth. The cancer also produces molecules that break down the barriers formed by healthy cells, allowing the cancer to infiltrate surrounding tissues.

So, in treating cancer, we have a range of problems to tackle. There is uncontrolled proliferation of cells; and malignant cells' failure to commit suicide. On top of that, we have the formation of new blood vessels – a process called angiogenesis – and invasive spread. Each of these processes is controlled by specific molecules. And each of these molecules is a target for anti-cancer drugs.

When I started writing about cancer, the most important systemic treatments were various kinds of chemotherapy – drugs called cytotoxics, because they poisoned cells. Their poisonous effect was felt more by rapidly dividing cells than by slowly dividing ones; so the drugs were to some extent selective for cancer. But cells whose healthy function also involves rapid division, such as those that make up the immune system and line the gut, were also hit. Cytotoxics were a blunderbuss.

The situation has now improved radically. Although different cancers produce different molecules that need to be countered, we have drugs that are truly specific in their effects, and that are relatively non-toxic. In the long path of drug development, there were some disappointing turns along the way. But then the wheel turned again, and ideas that had seemed to be dead-ends turned out – after all – to lead to successful outcomes. With cancer, we are talking Test Match cricket, and not T20.

The "abs" and the "ibs"

Most targeted anti-cancer agents block the growth-promoting molecular signals that are found around or within cancer cells. Certain drugs "mop up" growth factors circulating in the blood before they get a chance to bind to and activate growth receptors on cells (see Figure). Other drugs prevent growth factors gaining access to receptors by occupying them themselves, acting like a key that fits the lock but does not open the door. Then there are drugs that work within the cancer cell itself to block the transmission of messages from an activated growth receptor to the nucleus, so preventing the command to divide from being put into effect.

Drugs that act outside the cell or on its surface are often large molecule antibodies based on genetically engineered bits of our own immune system and are given intravenously. (So US oncologists still like them.) Their chemical names end in "ab". The first of these agents to prove life-saving in breast cancer was trastuzumab (Herceptin). Drugs that work within the cell are small molecules taken in tablet form. Their chemical names often end in "ib".

Imatinib (or Glivec) is a small molecule with a big place in medicine. A particular form of leukaemia called CML occurs when parts

Cancer: playing the long game

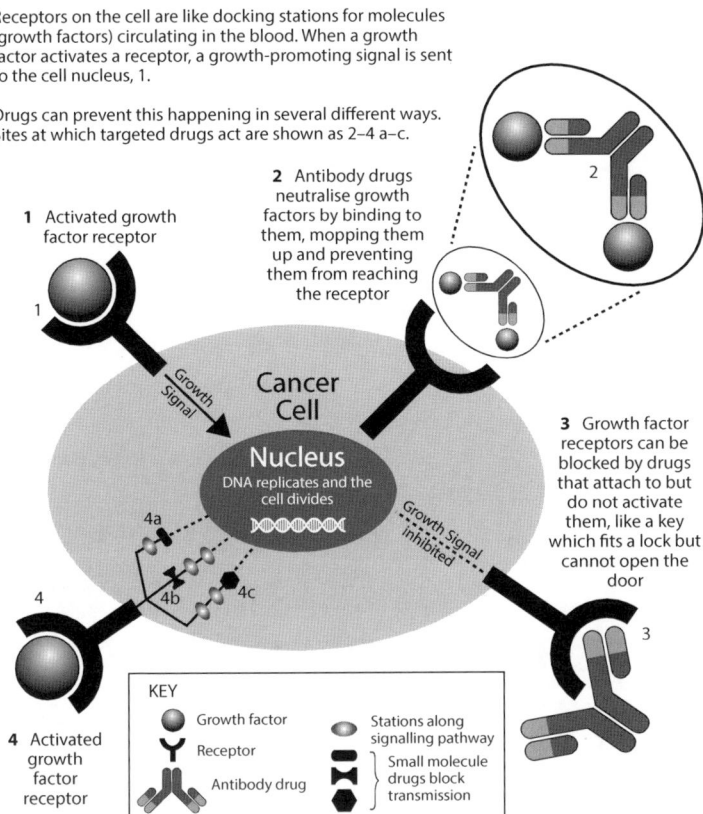

HOW TARGETED DRUGS WORK

Receptors on the cell are like docking stations for molecules (growth factors) circulating in the blood. When a growth factor activates a receptor, a growth-promoting signal is sent to the cell nucleus, 1.

Drugs can prevent this happening in several different ways. Sites at which targeted drugs act are shown as 2–4 a–c.

1 Activated growth factor receptor

2 Antibody drugs neutralise growth factors by binding to them, mopping them up and preventing them from reaching the receptor

3 Growth factor receptors can be blocked by drugs that attach to but do not activate them, like a key which fits a lock but cannot open the door

4 Activated growth factor receptor

KEY: Growth factor, Receptor, Antibody drug, Stations along signalling pathway, Small molecule drugs block transmission

of two chromosomes become switched. Cells with this abnormality produce a protein which causes them to grow out of control. Imatinib was designed specifically to target the underlying mutation and has extended for many years the lives of people with CML.

This was a lucky break, since the problem causing CML was relatively easy to tackle. More often, a growth signal has several paths it can follow to reach the nucleus and activate cell division.

As with the London Underground, you can find one station blocked and find a way to your destination using alternative routes. So we need to give drugs that block several pathways at once. Devising combinations of targeted agents that achieve this is now a big challenge for cancer specialists.

Since five or so years ago, we have also had have several immunomodulator drugs that increase the life expectancy of patients with cancers – among others – of the kidney, lung and colon, and melanoma by "taking the brakes off" our bodies' own immune response to tumours.

These advances have come through extraordinarily diligent effort, and after many disappointments. "Cloning a killer for the front line against cancer" was the headline of a piece I wrote in 1984 for the *Futures* page of *The Guardian*. Ten years later I had to follow it up with another piece – explaining why the high hopes of this breakthrough, as with several others, had not been fulfilled – which a witty subeditor titled "Sense of tumour failure".

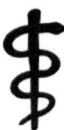

CLONING A KILLER FOR THE FRONT LINE

The Guardian December 1984

In the fight to find a drug to destroy cancer cells, researchers are hopeful that American genetic engineers have produced a natural substance that can attack malignant disease.

Cloning a killer for the front line

To compensate for the fading promise of other "breakthroughs", we now have two new, potent, natural killers of cancer cells, and there is hope that these products of our own immune system can be harnessed in the fight against malignancies.

Bioengineers at Genentech have now cloned the human genes that code for tumour necrosis factor (TNF) and lymphotoxin. This means both proteins can be harvested in quantities large enough to allow treatment of patients on a trial basis. Genentech's initial experiments in San Francisco show the pure, genetically engineered factors are effective against tumours in animals. Still – after recent disappointments – can we be confident their two new substances will eventually find a place in therapy?

Karol Sikora, director of the Ludwig Institute for Cancer Research in Cambridge, has been sceptical about the practical value of other recent discoveries. "There's been an awful lot of hype", he says. "But, if anything significant is going to come out of the 1980s, tumour necrosis factor will be it."

"Wonder drug" is a formidable tag to hang on any molecule. Since penicillin, none has lived up to it. And the cloning of TNF is not going to do for cancer what Alexander Fleming's contaminated dish did for the treatment of bacterial infections. But TNF starts with several advantages.

It is one or two hundred times more potent a killer of tumour cells than interferon. It is also more selective, so normal cells are less at risk. And it can probably be given by injections so that it will circulate throughout the body.

Cancer cells become dispersed, giving rise to tumour

colonies wherever they settle. It is often this secondary spread of the disease, rather than the primary tumour, which leads to death. In practice, it means that any really effective remedy will have to follow tumour cells into every corner of the body. Treatment must be "systemic". Radiotherapy and surgery alone – which can only treat small areas of tissue – cannot cure advanced disease.

Another major difficulty is that tumour cells are in most ways very similar to the healthy counterparts from which they derive. Present drugs do not recognise the small differences that exist.

The model to emulate is the body's own immune system. Elements within it can both identify tumour cells and produce substances that kill them. If we could dissect out either the recognition or the tumoricidal elements, beef them up a bit, and then put them back into the body, we would be far further along the road to curing cancer.

Fuss has been made about the lymphokines, of which interleukin-2 is an example, but they are molecules involved in enabling immune system cells to "talk" to each other. They are not at the sharp end of the system. Tumour necrosis factor and lymphotoxin are far more exciting since these molecules are actually in the business of killing tumour cells.

Interest in the anti-cancer toxins began in 1891, when the New York physician William Coley noted that tumours shrank in some patients who had severe bacterial infections. It was not the bacterial toxin itself that killed cancer cells, but something the body produced in response to it. The substance was termed Tumour Necrosis Factor, or TNF.

It became clear that TNF was produced by wandering white blood cells, or macrophages, of the kind that we know infiltrate tumours. But it was not possible to get enough TNF to work out its structure, and it could not be concentrated and purified.

The Genentech work is crucial because the DNA blueprint that codes for human TNF has now been isolated and cloned in bacteria. For the first time, the pure substance can be harvested in sufficient quantities from the bacterial production line for it to be used in clinical trials. Already, cloned recombinant TNF has been used in animals with cancers implanted under the skin, producing significant shrinkage.

Genentech has a good track record. In 1980 they were the first to clone the interferon gene and start producing the substance in its pure form. More impressive still, the cloning of TNF is only half of the double first announced in this week's issue of *Nature*, since Genentech have pulled off the same trick with lymphotoxin.

Postscript

In the early 1980s, the buzz was in "biological response modifiers". We were going to dissect out elements of the immune response, amplify them, and set them to work on tumours with devastating effect. It came to very little [see below]: interleukins, interferons, and even tumour necrosis factor proved sadly ineffective against the most common tumours (breast, lung, prostate, colon) and were unexpectedly toxic when given in pharmacological doses.

We had to wait until the new millennium brought understanding of the gene mutations driving cancers – and the development of drugs to target them – before we had radically new systemic therapies. But that did not mean the 1980s and 1990s were devoid of progress.

In the mid 1980s, the ball-park cure rate for cancer overall was about 50%. (Cure in this context was conventionally taken as meaning alive five years after diagnosis.) In 2006, the United States Centers for Disease Control estimated a cure rate of around 65% for people diagnosed with cancer in the years 1997–2002.

The improvement in this period was due to earlier diagnosis, better surgery, better radiotherapy, better hormone and chemotherapy and better supportive care. A big part of this success was in breast cancer. This was achieved by treating women after surgery – even if they had no obvious signs of cancer – with the anti-oestrogen agent tamoxifen. Although it came initially from a research programme in contraception at ICI's labs in Alderley Park, Cheshire, tamoxifen was developed as a cancer drug in the 1980s. Its oestrogen-blocking effect reduces the chances that microscopic cancers will become life-threatening recurrences and so cuts the chances of dying from breast cancer over the next five to fifteen years by 10–15 percent. Since breast cancer is such a common disease, the number of lives saved worldwide amounts to millions. Tamoxifen is one of the most important drugs ever developed.

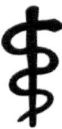

Sense of tumour failure

The Guardian June 1996

More than a decade ago, scientists made what they assumed were two major advances. First, they identified substances which they thought formed the body's front-line defence against cancer and engineered bacteria to produce them in quantities large enough to be given to patients.

Secondly, they developed techniques to manufacture the antibodies which could be used to *label* malignant cells. So, in theory, even conventional anti-cancer drugs could be delivered directly to tumours, bypassing toxicity to healthy tissues.

Our bodies are capable of killing cancer cells. But in the past decade we have failed to make reliable allies of these anti-cancer defences.

Tumour Necrosis Factor (TNF) offered the greatest hope [see above]. But it turned out to be "a complete bust", according to Karol Sikora, professor of clinical oncology at London's Hammersmith Hospital. In the 1980s, a thousand cancer patients were given TNF with no success at all. Far from being a cancer killer, certain tumours actually secrete TNF themselves.

Interferon and interleukin-2, also involved in the body's anti-tumour response, have fared only slightly better. They benefit patients with certain blood and kidney cancers, but together these make up less than two percent of all cancers. Neither agent is active against the major killers, cancers of the lung, breast and colon.

"Interferon and interleukin reset the immune system, and certain rare cancers happen to be susceptible to immune attack. But the common cancers are not," says Karol Sikora.

Dr Frances Balkwill, head of biological therapies for the Imperial Cancer Research Fund, worked on interferon. Along with the media, there were scientists who over-interpreted the early evidence, she admits. "It was very optimistic to expect interferon to cure large cancers. It worked in animals, but only when there was little tumour present," she recalls. "Yet interferon was given first to patients with advanced disease."

Doctors set the biological agents too hard a task too early. But they also massively underestimated the complexity of the systems they were dealing with. It is now clear there are dozens of different molecules, each playing a subtly different role. "These substances are communication molecules which allow cells to talk to each other, but even now we don't know what language they are speaking," says Karol Sikora.

There was also an important misconception from the start about how these agents might work. In the natural situation, interferon and interleukin affect only a small number of cells around the ones that secrete them. They are not designed to circulate round the body. Yet the only practical means of giving these substances is by injection. Used in this way they stimulate release of a raft of other biological agents, with effects that are near impossible to predict and control.

Even at low doses, interferon produces flu-like symptoms. In high doses it puts patients into a coma. "TNF is highly toxic," Dr Balkwill explains. "But it was unlucky that the maximum dose tolerated by man turns out to be one fortieth of that tolerated by mice."

Monoclonal antibodies have also proved disappointing. Of the "magic bullet" antibodies which were to deliver chemical toxins or radioactivity direct to tumour cells, only one – a follow up to surgery for bowel cancer – is in clinical use.

The concept now is one of keeping cancer at bay, says Dr Balkwill. "The idea that you could treat it like an ear infection with the equivalent of an antibiotic has gone."

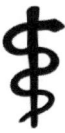

In his short story *Unprofessional*, published in 1932, Rudyard Kipling writes of how watching cells around the clock under a microscope reveals biological "tides" that differ between healthy and cancerous tissues; and he has one of his characters speculate that cancer surgery might achieve a better outcome if timed accordingly.

The idea that chemotherapy might also be optimised by following circadian rhythms – chronotherapy – is elegant and plausible but has never become mainstream. At one point, though, it looked as if the tide was running in its favour.

COUNTING ON THE CANCER CLOCK

The Guardian December 1987

Evidence to be presented at a cancer specialists' meeting in Dallas, Texas, will suggest that giving cancer drugs at times dictated by the body's daily rhythms improves their effectiveness and reduces the risk of side-effects.

Dr Francis Levi, director of the Laboratory of Biological Rhythms and Chronotherapy, and one of France's leading researchers [he later moved to the University of Warwick], offers two explanations for this remarkable effect. One is that the body's healthy cells vary through the day in their ability to tolerate anti-cancer drugs. This means that precise timing enables a higher dose of drug to be given without severe side-effects. The other is that tumour cells also have their own daily cycles of sensitivity and resistance.

The specialists will hear the results of a French study of almost 200 patients with bowel cancer which had spread, a condition that is notoriously hard to treat. One group was given continuous infusion of drugs for five days. The other received the drugs only at carefully chosen times of the day and night.

The tumour shrank to less than half its original size in 50 per cent of patients who had drug therapy adjusted to biological rhythms. But the cancer responded in only 30 per cent of the patients given the drugs at a constant rate.

The idea that drug treatment can be adjusted to fit in with the rhythms of our internal biological clock is not new, but the French study is the best evidence yet that the idea can work. The trial involved two highly toxic cancer drugs, 5-FU and a platinum compound, and was based on experiments conducted ten years ago on mice and rats, which showed that 5-FU caused least damage to healthy animals when given in the middle of the day, while platinum toxicity was at its lowest when the drug was delivered at 4am.

Since rodents have a sleep and waking cycle that is the reverse of ours, Dr Levi reversed the timings for his human patients. The 5-FU was given in the middle of the night and platinum in the middle of the day. "We arranged that the delivery of 5-FU would gradually increase over six hours, reaching a maximum at 4am, followed by a gradual reduction. The reverse pattern was followed with platinum," Dr Levi says.

It is too early to say how long the new treatment will keep patients free of disease symptoms, but there is a trend towards longer disease-free survival. Dr Levi believes that one reason for the greater effect of treatment is that patients were able to take the anti-cancer drugs as planned, without the need for doses to be reduced or delayed. Far fewer of his patients on chronotherapy suffered serious mouth ulcers or loss of sensation in the fingers and feet, the two side-effects that normally limit the amount of drugs that can be given.

But another possibility is that tumour cells also have a daily cycle of activity that makes them more sensitive to drugs given at certain times, particularly during the night, because that is when they are most likely to divide.

Such cycles have not yet been identified in bowel cancer cells. But they have been seen in cancers of the ovary, lymphatic system and head and neck.

Dr Bill Hrushesky, a senior cancer specialist at the Stratton Veterans' Administration Centre in Albany, New York, is another key figure in chronotherapy. In the eighties, he studied the effect of giving drugs at specific times of the day to women with ovarian cancer. The evidence was that the precise timing of treatment could affect survival.

In the trial, half the patients were given one drug at 6am and another at 6pm. In the other group, the regime was reversed. In the first group, 44 per cent of women were alive after five years, while in the second group only 11 per cent remained.

He also draws attention to the daily rhythms in the release of many of our hormones, such as cortisol and melatonin. The particular level of one or more of these hormones may influence the anti- cancer effect of drugs.

Finally, there is a daily cycle in the state of activation of the immune system. "At certain times it may be easier to stimulate it into attacking cancer cells that have been damaged but not yet killed by anti-cancer drugs," he argues. "Each of these four factors is already known to be relevant to the response of cancer to treatment."

At Dr Hrushesky's hospital, drug regimes varied according to time of day are now in routine use for cancer patients. And he believes that the importance of chronotherapy can only increase.

Postscript

Marc Lippman, of the US National Cancer Institute, developed a way of using oestrogen to bring breast cancer cells into their most susceptible state before giving chemotherapy. By his analogy, this is like lining horses up in the starting gate and then firing a single bullet through their heads. (Terrible diseases breed violent metaphors.) All our cells – healthy and cancerous – follow daily cycles; and the idea of finding a sweet point when healthy cells are at their most resistant to toxic drugs while cancer cells are at their most susceptible is a neat idea. But its time has not yet come; and perhaps it never will.

Chapter Eleven

Danger: doctors at work

Well into the 1970s, many consultants held to the idea that forcing junior doctors to work punishingly long hours was almost a rite of passage: we had had to experience it, so why shouldn't they? There was also the view that long hours were needed to fully learn the trade.

World Medicine September 1980

At 3.30 in the afternoon of February 17th 1976, Dr Chattur left a Gateshead hospital to drive the few miles to his home in Newcastle. Minutes later he fell asleep at the wheel of his car and crashed, sustaining fatal injuries. Apart from a two-hour break for breakfast, Dr Chattur had been working continuously for 31 hours and had lost a full night's sleep.

Dr Chattur's colleagues complained bitterly that he and four others had been sharing the workload of eight anaesthetists. They said that long hours were usual and such an accident almost inevitable. The British Medical Association took up the case and obtained a larger pension for Dr Chattur's family under the NHS regulation governing compensation for injuries at work.

Such cases are rare but highlight problems caused by loss of sleep that are likely to affect the wellbeing of doctor and patient alike. If Dr Chattur's fatigue made him unable to stay awake driving home in mid-afternoon, he might equally well have fallen asleep in the operating theatre. How can we be happy about the judgment of people suffering to this extent from exhaustion?

In June [1980], the BMA released the results of a survey showing that 27 percent of junior doctors worked more than a hundred hours a week, and 70 percent more than eighty hours. In a study of 2500 doctors in 1973, 40 percent said their long hours on duty often or always impaired their ability to work. This is hardly surprising: in the 24 hours before the survey, they had spent an average of eight hours on call and 13 hours at work. Many indicated that the periods when they were most tired coincided with those when they had least supervision.

Two experiments relate directly to the kind of tasks doctors are routinely required to perform. A paper in the *New England Journal* in 1971 reported a study of 15 New York doctors who were given a twenty minute ECG recording and asked to mark episodes of cardiac arrhythmia. Each doctor was studied once when fatigued (having averaged 1.8 hours of sleep in the previous 32) and once after they had slept for seven hours. Doctors made nearly twice as many errors when they were short of sleep – and this was despite the motivation provided by the offer of a $75 prize.

A second study, carried out at Addenbrooke's Hospital in Cambridge and published in the journal *Ergonomics* in 1978, points in the same direction. Researchers spent a month studying junior doctors' grammatical reasoning and ability to understand lab test results, and related their performance to extent of fatigue. Three hours of lost sleep was sufficient to reduce scores on the logical reasoning task. It was not enough to affect the doctors' ability to identify grossly abnormal readings in the haematology and blood chemistry reports.

And, paradoxically, 4–5 hours' lost sleep actually improved performance on this task. But, after they had lost 7–8 hours, there was marked deterioration.

Sleep loss and disruption

The wider literature on sleep shows the true state of fatigue induced by one night's total deprivation: half of us will fall asleep within one minute of closing our eyes. It also shows that sleep deprivation reduces our willingness to put effort into work. In research from Sweden, subjects were asked to do arithmetic reasoning tasks. One group was told that certain items were insoluble while the other was not. When sleep-deprived, subjects who had been given an "excuse" for failure left more items unsolved and spent less time on task than after normal sleep.

Repeatedly losing part of a night's sleep can have effects as great as total sleep deprivation, as shown by a six-week experiment run by Bob Wilkinson at the MRC Applied Psychology Unit in Cambridge in which a group of naval ratings were subjected to two-day periods of varying sleep loss. After the first night, performance deteriorated only if the sailors had had two hours or less sleep but, after the second night, poorer performance was apparent even if they had slept for five hours.

How long does it take to recover? Bob Wilkinson estimates that most people sleep nine to twelve hours after a period of prolonged wakefulness. This recovery sleep does not replace lost sleep hour for hour. The compensatory mechanism seems to be an increase in the proportion of time spent in the deepest (slow-wave) stages of sleep.

If this period of recovery is curtailed, the effects of sleep loss persist. Akerstedt and Gillberg, of the Stockholm Stress Research Lab, were impressed by the bizarre effects obtained when people were woken during recovery sleep. Subjects seemed confused, were often unable to recollect events, and would sometimes deny they had been woken at all. Doctors sometimes complain they cannot remember phone calls which have woken them after a long period on duty. More disturbing still, they occasionally cannot remember decisions they made in response.

To the extent that a doctor's work is generally varied, interesting, and played for high stakes, the effects of sleep loss will be minimised. But, since doctors experience a combination of acute sleep loss and chronic disturbance of sleep, the effects of each will be potentiated.

As the period of sleep loss, irregularity, and disturbance increases, it becomes impossible to prevent momentary lapses of consciousness. Donald Broadbent, for many years head of the Cambridge Applied Psychology Unit, uses an analogy to describe these microsleeps. We are not like a child's mechanical toy which goes slower as it runs down. Nor are we like a car engine which runs normally until its tank is empty. We are more like a motor which, after much use, misfires, runs normally for a while, and then falters again.

It was presumably just such a faltering which was responsible for Dr Chattur's fatal crash. With present hours of work, it is a wonder that similar and equally tragic events do not occur more often.

Postscript

Tragedies did continue. For example, in 1994, a doctor working at St Bartholomew's Hospital in Rochester, Kent – who had had four hours' broken sleep during a 34-hour shift – misread a label and wrongly administered the cancer drug vincristine, killing a sixty year old man with leukaemia.

European Union regulations designed to limit long hours for all workers eventually enforced change. In the UK, Working Time Regulations introduced in 1998 applied fully to junior doctors from 2009. The limit is 48 hours work per week averaged across 26 weeks. But a large survey published in the *British Medical Journal* in 2014 found that the relationship between trainee and senior doctors meant that many juniors still felt required to work longer hours "voluntarily".

Chapter Twelve

A fertile furrow

Although in origin a programme about farming, *The Archers* has always been rich in medical interest and incident.

A SERIES OF UNFORTUNATE EVENTS? MORTALITY IN A BORSETSHIRE VILLAGE

British Medical Journal Christmas issue, December 2011

The mortality rate for characters in the television soap operas *Coronation Street* and *EastEnders* exceeds those of bomb disposal experts and racing drivers. Many deaths are violent, and the overall five year survival of recently introduced characters is poorer than that for many cancers. Does the same dramatic imperative lead the long running BBC radio series *The Archers* to contain a similarly high level of mortality? Or does radio, and the bucolic setting, give everyday country folk a better chance in life?

The village of Ambridge is set in a rural area south of Birmingham. Among the population of 700, employment in farming is higher than average but the age distribution is similar to the rest of the country, with 20% aged under 16 years and 20% aged 65 and over.

We are directly acquainted with 60 inhabitants but have knowledge of a further 55, giving a total – for epidemiological purposes – of 115 (58 men and 57 women). In such a

A series of unfortunate events?

Deaths by cause September 1992 to September 2011 among Ambridge population of whom we are aware (n=115)

Type of death	Year	Name	Age (years)	Cause or circumstance of death
Accident	1994	Mark Hebden	38	Road traffic accident
	1998	John Archer	22	Tractor overturned
	2011	Nigel Pargetter*	51	Fall from roof
Suicide	2004	Greg Turner	41	Self inflicted gunshot wound
Heart attack (confirmed)	1996	Martha Woodford	73	Heart attack
	1996	Guy Pemberton	65	Heart attack†
	2005	George Barford	76	Heart attack
	2005	Betty Tucker	55	Heart attack†
	2010	Sid Perks*	65	Heart attack
Presumed heart attack	2005	Julia Pargetter	81	Died in her sleep
	2010	Phil Archer	81	Found dead in armchair
Cancer	1996	Irene Barraclough	76	Site of tumour not specified
	2007	Siobhan Donovan née Hathaway*‡		Melanoma
Unexplained	1998	Tom Forrest‡		Died in care home
	1998	Pru Forrest‡		Died in care home six days after Tom

* Death did not occur in Ambridge itself.
† Having had non-fatal heart attack some weeks previously. ‡Siobhan was middle aged; both Tom and Pru were elderly.

small sample, few events of epidemiological significance are likely to occur in any given year. In calculating death rates, I therefore pooled data for the 20 years preceding the time of writing.

Of the 15 deaths, nine were of male characters and six of female characters. This equates to a mortality rate of 7.8 per 1000 population per year for males. For comparison, the mortality rate for England and Wales was 8.5 per 1000. For females, the mortality rate calculated from the Ambridge data is 5.2 deaths per 1000, and the comparable national rate is 5.8. Hence the overall mortality rate in Ambridge over the 20 years to September 2011 was marginally lower than that in the country as a whole.

That said, do the causes of death in and around Ambridge reflect wider experience? Among male Archers characters, the three accidental deaths and one suicide (27% of the total mortality) substantially over-represent the risk evident nationally. In 2000, accidents accounted for only 4% of deaths in men.

The five confirmed cardiac deaths account for 33% of total mortality in Ambridge (rising to 47% if two probable heart attacks are included). Yet cardiac deaths nationally in 2000 accounted for only 23% of mortality in males and 17% of that in females. In Ambridge, heart disease seems to have a particularly poor prognosis. (This would make sense for practical reasons, as the sudden death of characters is sometimes necessitated by the sudden death of the actors who portray them.)

In contrast to cardiac mortality, that due to cancer is under-represented. If the national pattern prevailed, cancers would account for roughly a quarter of deaths among characters. The two deaths observed (one from melanoma and the other from a malignancy of unspecified site) represent only 13% of the total.

To compensate for the 15 deaths in the past 20 years, 13 children have been born to the 115 characters. The annual live birth rate in Ambridge in 1992–2011 was 5.6 per 1000. In England and Wales in 2001 it was 11.4 per 1000. Notable among the births were those of Phoebe Aldridge in a tepee during the Glastonbury Festival and of the Pargetter twins. Two births were sufficiently premature to require the services of a neonatal intensive care unit, one of them due to pre-eclampsia.

Illness

In addition to the obstetric complications, Ambridge characters have experienced a range of life threatening accidental injuries and acute and chronic physical and psychiatric morbidity. For example, the Hebden family suffered further ill luck when Daniel developed juvenile arthritis, which has a prevalence of only 1–2 per thousand children. However, despite the poor prognosis associated with systemic onset below the age of five, the condition has fully resolved.

Ruth Archer's breast cancer was oestrogen receptor negative and multifocal, requiring mastectomy. She went on to have another child after adjuvant chemotherapy and is free of relapse at 10 years. No cases of colorectal, prostate, or lung cancer have occurred among the 115 characters followed since 1992. With the possible exception of Joe Grundy's dubious self diagnosis of farmer's lung, little respiratory disease has occurred.

A *foreign correspondent in medicine*

The medical histories of Ambridge characters illustrate well the series' interest in creating complex and slow burning story lines. Elizabeth Archer (born with congenital heart disease in 1967) had two early corrective procedures but more than 20 years later she had a valve replacement (after a twin pregnancy). Then, after a further decade, ventricular tachycardia led to implantation of a cardioverter-defibrillator in March 2011. (Nationally, fewer than 100 such implants were carried out in 2009, so she may have had privileged access to expensive devices.)

A significant lag may occur between the suggestion of a medical storyline and its use. John Wynn-Jones, a general practitioner advising the programme in 1992, identified depression and suicide as an aspect of rural life that could be covered. Greg Turner's illness and death occurred more than 10 years later.

A consequence of Greg Turner's suicide was mental health problems for Helen Archer, which were still being played out six years later. The way in which the slow but relentless unravelling of Jack Woolley's world has been portrayed over the six years since Alzheimer's disease was first suspected has been appreciated by critics.

With the exception of infidelity, nothing captures an audience more completely than death, a complicated birth, or an interesting illness. However, in the case of overall mortality over 20 years, *The Archers* – by luck or good editorial judgment – reflected almost exactly the experience of the wider population of England and Wales. In its rate of births, village life seemed less eventful than reproductive life nationally. The epidemiological features that seem to stand out as dramatically different from the norm are the poor survival after a heart attack and the high proportion of deaths due to accidental or self inflicted injury, which is sevenfold greater than that expected on the basis of national data.

In its higher than expected number of traumatic deaths, *The Archers* is similar to soap operas set in urban environments and on television. However, in overall mortality, which in epidemiological terms is the most important outcome, *The Archers* ploughs its own furrow. Is that the charm of the rural, or of radio?

Postscript

In the period 2012–2018, mortality rates for both men and women continued to be remarkably close to the national average. There has been one death from cancer, and one (Jack Woolley) from Alzheimer's; but the most unexpected, dramatic and tragic by far was Nic Grundy's death from sepsis in 2018.

The unusually high rate of deaths from accident or suicide is no longer evident. The same is true for cardiac deaths. Over the period 1992 to 2011, all seven heart attacks had been fatal. Yet, when Tony Archer had a heart attack in 2012, he survived. Since this was soon after the *British Medical Journal* article, I asked one of the production team if my paper had saved Tony's life. Her reply was: "What power! Fun, isn't it?"

A follow-up piece for the *Times* (written with Chris Smyth) looked at events of sociological rather than medical significance.

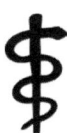

Sex, scandal, crime ... Ambridge is just following national trends

The Times August 2013

The steamy start of an affair between Helen Archer and the mega-dairy manager Rob Titchener has again prompted complaints about sensation-seeking on *The Archers*. The appointment of an editor who has previously worked on *Footballers' Wives* and *Hollyoaks* only heightened fears of sexing up on the soap.

Analysis reveals, however, that the series really is an everyday story of country folk. Rates of divorce, births out of wedlock and sexual assault in Ambridge have kept pace with national statistics and may even be lower than in reality. When the series began 63 years ago, characters such as Dan and Doris Archer lived lives of blameless rectitude, as befitted a country where divorce and illegitimacy were still scandalous.

A search through the *Archers* archives shows that since then Ambridge – as one might expect from a quiet rural community – has followed rather than led social trends. Today, among the 70 residents with speaking parts, there have been nine divorces. This seems tame compared with the 40% of marriages nationally which end in divorce.

Elizabeth Archer had an abortion in 1992 but since then there has been just one more, when Annette Turner decided not to have the baby of Leon, the Australian barman. National figures suggest that over the past twenty years we would expect seven terminations among twenty women of childbearing age.

In 1967, the birth of Jennifer Aldridge's illegitimate child, Adam, divided the nation at a time when only seven children in a hundred were born out of wedlock. Forty years later, when Jennifer (now Aldridge) agreed to raise Ruairi, love child of her husband, Brian, the drama gripped the audience but the fact that he was born to a couple who were not married was no longer cause for comment. Ruairi was in the same position as 45% of children.

When Adam Macy and Ian Craig entered into a civil partnership in 2006, it made headlines. But, among 110 known characters, a single gay wedding makes Ambridge pretty average. The rape of Kathy Perks in 2005 again prompted accusations that Ambridge was turning into Albert Square. But such an attack has not been repeated and, taking the current national average of one serious sexual offence per thousand of the population per year, we might have expected at least one more case over the past twenty years.

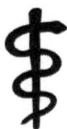

Doctor with his finger on Ambridge's pulse

The Independent March 1992

The Archers will receive a dose of preventive medicine, thanks to the arrival of a GP adviser.

A foreign correspondent in medicine

True *Archers* buffs will not have missed the intriguing subplot developing around Elizabeth's recent bouts of nausea. Could it be morning sickness, perhaps, or something less portentous? Illness makes almost as compelling drama as infidelity, and infirmities of one form or another have always had a place in Radio 4's flagship soap opera.

Now, Dr John Wynn-Jones, from the rural Welsh Marches, has joined the programme's production team as its first general practice adviser. He is keen to add a leavening of health promotion to the mix of Ambridge medicine.

The influence of soaps on ideas about illness should not be underestimated. The depression suffered by Mike Tucker, the failed Ambridge farmer, will probably have done more than the Royal College of Psychiatrists to inform the nation that not everyone with mental problems thinks they are Napoleon. One early result of Dr Wynn-Jones' influence is the appearance of the community psychiatric nurse who is helping Mike Tucker. Dr Wynn-Jones argues that this group of health professionals has done as much as any to improve care in his own community.

Because of this enlightened approach to psychiatric illness, there is now a queue of medical charities wanting their concerns to be featured on the programme. Vanessa Whitburn, who runs *The Archers* from the BBC's Pebble Mill studios in Birmingham, is used to such approaches. Would it be possible to feature an Ambridge child with Down's syndrome or dyslexia? What about breast cancer, or has that been done too recently by *Brookside*? [see postscript]

Most suggestions are rejected because introducing difficult medical conditions can be fraught with problems. Ms Whitburn says: "A successful story is slow-burning, psychologically and clinically. It is accepted only if everyone feels strongly that it fits the character concerned."

There is clearly a limit to the number of illnesses the 48-strong cast can contract. But in this microcosm of epidemiology, we would have expected a terminal chronic disease or two before now. Four years ago, there was a teaser which suggested the programme was heading in that direction. However, Kenton Archer's ill-defined malaise, widely suspected of presaging AIDS, turned out to be caused by an underactive thyroid. The diagnostic acumen of Matthew Thorogood, the Ambridge GP, was called into question: given that Kenton's Mum had the same condition, he might have spotted it sooner. But the audience had to be hooked, and no-one really minded being kidded.

To its credit, the programme has not shunned controversy. When it turned out that Phil Archer's hip replacement would have to be done privately because of the two-year NHS wait, William Waldegrave, the health secretary, was not amused and told Ms Whitburn so when they met at an Enuresis Society function. (Bedwetting had featured 10 months previously, with Emma Carter, six, as the sufferer.)

But Mr Waldegrave had to be satisfied with the BBC researchers' impeccable plot preparation. Three hospitals – Redditch, Worcester and Wolverhampton – which served Ambridge's notional part of Worcestershire had been contacted and none could have done the operation sooner.

Although storyline development is the responsibility of the production team, there are eight expert advisers with briefs ranging from religion to agriculture. The programme also takes advice from a hospital doctor. But Dr Wynn-Jones may have significant influence. He took on the unpaid job of

GP adviser after approaching Ms Whitburn too talk about how general practice could be better promoted.

After 12 years as a GP in Montgomery, he is particularly interested in health problems affecting rural communities: social isolation and economic decline lead to stress and potential suicide, there is under-reporting of farm accidents, and the ever-present threat of humans catching animal diseases. "Medicine in *The Archers* so far has followed a disease model, not a health model," Dr Wynn-Jones says. "Though young, Matthew Thorogood is an old-style GP, reacting to illness and not trying to prevent it."

When he moves south, as he soon will, there will be fresh opportunities. It is likely the new doctor will be trying to make farmers aware of organisms in their livestock responsible for infection, and tightening up on accident prevention. "Just think of the Grundy children, growing up without the protection of the Health and Safety Act," Dr Wynn-Jones laments.

Postscript

Bethany, who has Down's syndrome, was born to Vicky and Mike Tucker in 2013. Ruth Archer developed breast cancer in 2000 and has been successfully treated with surgery and adjuvant chemotherapy. Greg Turner, gamekeeper, committed suicide in 2004.

Chapter Thirteen

A long view of the gut

POETRY IN MOTION

Pharmacy Update February 1986

Big stools are beautiful, according to Dr Denis Burkitt's ideal of defecation, and they are especially to be admired when of cowpat consistency with a little cone on top. Dr Burkitt is a man overwhelmingly concerned for the quantity and quality of the nation's motions: and he is not shy about saying so. Fortunately, bowels are second only to the weather as a favoured topic of conversation, he believes. Hence there is ample opportunity for dispensing advice on the role of fibre in increasing stool bulk and promoting health and happiness.

"Problem number one", says Denis Burkitt, "Is that by world standards we are a totally constipated country. The USA is also totally constipated – from coast to coast. Lack of fibre is the fundamental cause." The result is a rate of colon cancer eight times that in rural Africa. And that is not the only medical problem caused by too little fibre. There is appendicitis, hiatus hernia, and diabetes; half our population suffers at some time from haemorrhoids; large numbers of women over the age of forty have varicose veins; and one in three of us develops gallstones.

All are diseases attributable to an over-processed diet. Fibre-depleted foods also make us fat. A few years ago, we didn't understrnand fibre, just as we didn't understand tonsils. The reaction was "cut it out."

As well as diseases obviously related to the gastrointestinal tract, and others caused by straining at stool, lack of fibre is emerging as a risk factor in breast cancer. There is good experimental evidence that fat is implicated, and straws in the wind suggesting a protective role for fibre. From Tufts University comes research showing that vegetarians get a third less breast cancer than non-vegetarians. There is evidence that more oestrogens are excreted as stool mass increases. And a Californian study of aspirate from nipples shows that the number of precancerous cells is related to the degree of constipation of the patient.

"Overall", Dr Burkitt says, "The amount of stool passed daily is a better indication of health than blood lipids, or glucose test, or chest X-ray. Life insurance companies need measure nothing else."

The equation is simple: low fibre equals small stools equals large hospitals. High fibre equals large stools equals small hospitals.

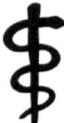

CAN YOU CATCH AN ULCER?

New Scientist May 1990

A bacterium may be an important cause of stomach and duodenal ulcers, and possibly of gastric cancer.

The pathogen, of the Helicobacter family, is able to survive in acidic conditions because it makes its own neutralisng alkali. By doing that, it tricks the stomach into upping its acid production.

Kenneth McColl, consultant gastroenterologist at Glasgow's Western Infirmary, has studied the effect of the bacterium in people and thinks the organism's ability to neutralise acid may be at the root of its ability to cause disease.

Duodenal ulcers are common, can be healed initially, but almost invariably relapse. Doctors believe that they arise when the stomach produces too much gastric acid. Some researchers have suggested that stress or diet are part of the cause of this increased acid production, but there is no convincing evidence that they are involved.

In the past decade, clinical trials have demonstrated that an important reason duodenal ulcers return is the bacterium *Helicobacter pylori*, which infects the walls of the lower stomach, or antrum. The bacterium can survive despite the fact that the stomach's acidity kills all but the toughest microorganisms since it neutralises the acid by converting urea in gastric juice into alkaline ammonia.

The antrum produces the hormone gastrin, which stimulates the stomach to secrete acid. When the acidity peaks, the cells that produce gastrin are switched off. McColl says that by generating ammonia the bacterium deceives these gastrin-producing cells into thinking the stomach is less acidic than it is, so they go on making gastrin.

McColl and his colleagues treated people with *H. pylori* by giving them a cocktail of antibiotics and a bismuth compound. Curiously, bismuth was a part of the treatment doctors used for stomach complaints at the turn of the century. This eradicated the bacteria, and, without them, the stomach became less acidic. Earlier clinical trials showed that people given a short-term treatment that killed *H. pylori* remained free from duodenal ulcers for long periods. This treatment is more effective than using drugs that simply stop the acid being produced.

H. pylori spreads from one person to another by close contact, according to a recent study from Toronto. Brendan Drumm and his colleagues at the Hospital for Sick Children of the University of Toronto investigated the families of children who were suffering from gastritis, an inflammation of the stomach, caused by the bacteria.

They found that the children's brothers and sisters were far more likely to harbour the bacterium than other children chosen at random. So, too, were the children's mothers – though not their fathers. According to Drumm, the clustering of infection within families suggests that the bacteria spread from one person to another.

Researchers are also focusing on the possibility that *H. pylori* is a cause of stomach cancer. Scientists from the Imperial Cancer Research Fund's Cancer Epidemiology Unit in Oxford have compared levels of gastric cancer with the prevalence of *H. pylori* infection in different parts of China. They find that areas with high levels of the disease also have high levels of the bacterium.

The Oxford epidemiologists say that many factors over several decades affect the development of stomach tumours, and *H. pylori* may be one of them. They have studied people from Caerphilly, in South Wales, which has a high rate of gastric cancer. It also has high levels of *H. pylori*. About half of the elderly population harboured the bacterium, the great majority without ill effect. But there is a possible role for *H. pylori* in causing the cancer, the researchers say.

Active gastritis caused by heliobacter leads, in a small proportion of people, to atrophic gastritis, in which secreting glands in the stomach wall die off, causing a drop in production of acid. This allows bacteria which are not usually found in the stomach to flourish. The researchers believe that certain of these organisms convert nitrates into nitrites, which can cause cancer. If bacteria damage the layer of mucus which protects the stomach lining, it may make it easier for all manner of cancer-causing substances to enter.

Postscript

In 2005, Australian researchers Barry Marshall and Robin Warren were awarded a Nobel prize for their work establishing the role of *Helicobacter pylori* in causing gastritis and peptic ulcer disease (peptic ulcers are called gastric if they appear in the stomach and duodenal if they are in the first part of the small intestine). A key step in proving the link occurred in 1984 when Marshall drank a solution containing *H. pylori*. His self infection was quickly followed by the development of gastritis, and the bacterium was cultured from a biopsy of the inflamed tissue taken from his stomach. Dr Marshall then cured his condition with antibiotics.

Such evidence slowly convinced a medical establishment that did not believe bacteria could survive in the stomach and overcame the strategy of ignoring the story adopted by pharmaceutical companies who produced drugs to block stomach acid secretion.

Chapter Fourteen

From Virginia to vaping

When Oxford Dictionaries made "vape" their 2014 word of the year, the first recorded use they could find was in articles I wrote for *New Society* and *The Guardian* in 1983. I mention this to establish that I've long had an interest in nicotine, smoking and alternative means of nicotine administration, and the machinations of the tobacco industry.

From 1978 to 1984, I was working (at Newcastle and Cambridge Universities) on efforts to reduce the harm from cigarettes in people who could not or chose not to quit. We were trying to cut smokers' exposure to tar and carbon monoxide, while still providing enough nicotine for cigarettes to be acceptable.

This was consistent with government policies of the time. All over the world, health agencies were producing league tables that ranked available brands according to the amount of tar they produced. The tables were based on values obtained from the standardised smoking of cigarettes by machines. It soon became clear, though, that people did not behave like machines. Faced with a cigarette of reduced nicotine strength, smokers took more and deeper puffs, and left less unsmoked tobacco in the cigarette butt.

To my mind, there is a case for arguing that the cigarette manufacturers were also cheating the smoking machines. (This has clear parallels with the current scandal of car manufacturers and exhaust emissions.)

Probably the most effective means of reducing the smoke delivered by a cigarette, and so its delivery of tar, is to put small ventilation holes just above the filter. When a machine puffs on a cigarette, the smoke is diluted with a stream of air drawn through these tiny perforations. But when *people* are smoking, the two fingers holding the cigarette block many of the ventilation holes. I suspect that this was not an accidental aspect of design. I believe manufacturers also manipulated officially measured tar yields by playing around with the length of the cork-coloured tipping paper that influences the amount of unsmoked tobacco left in the butt.

Writing about these issues in 1981 earned me a rebuke from British American Tobacco's Dr M Oldman who – in an internal memo released, along with almost 50 million pages of tobacco industry documents, as a result of litigation in the US – described my article as "typical opportunistic journalism".

My work at the medical schools in Newcastle and Cambridge was funded by tobacco companies, and this was publicly acknowledged. The manufacturers were legitimately interested in how smokers responded to cigarettes delivering different amounts of tar and nicotine – which they produced to specifications that were jointly agreed with researchers.

But there are two interesting (and I think I previously untold) stories to explore here. One is how the government's well-intentioned strategy of encouraging smokers to switch to cigarettes of reduced tar delivery was far less effective than they hoped. The low tar road was almost as likely to lead to a premature dead end as the high road. And the other is about how the techniques used by cigarette manufacturers very likely undermined the strategy from the outset. We might even call this the great smoking machine swindle.

In the wider historical context, pursuit of the low-tar approach to cigarettes may have delayed the development of technologies that allowed intake of nicotine with zero accompanying tar – ie gum, patches and, above all vaping – which are a far more effective means of reducing the harm that arises from the nicotine habit. If smokers need something to suck, a substitute cigarette containing nicotine but little else seems like a good prospect – despite current concerns about vaping-induced lung injury (expressed, for example, in 2019 in the *New England Journal of Medicine*).

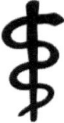

Homo fumens

World Medicine December 1978

In any prolonged "encounter of the third kind", attempts to explain the smoking habits of *Homo sapiens* would be an absorbing test of an extra-terrestrial anthropologist's wits. These bizarre acts of "smoke drinking", they might note, are irrelevant to the satisfaction of biological needs, play no part in religious or secular ritual, are regarded as slow-motion suicide even by adherents – and yet are practised by almost half of humanity across all barriers of race, class, politics and religion.

Baffled as they might be, the extraordinary thing is that if the extraterrestrials were in any way physiologically comparable with us, they would try smoking, probably overcome their initial revulsion, become confirmed smokers, and take the habit back to their home planet together with carefully preserved seedlings of *Nicotiana tabacum*.

The ubiquity of cigarette smoking and its persistence historically in the face of often rigorous proscription and, in our own times, despite agreed and severe health risks, is a remarkable phenomenon.

The many different forms which smoking takes and the complexity of the smoking act itself make it difficult to devise any unitary account of the behaviour and the rewards it offers. Image and status are probably important to cigar smokers, for example; aroma, taste and manipulative satisfactions perhaps paramount for the pipe smoker. It is also probable that the factors initiating smoking (curiosity, initiation, peer pressure, anticipation of adulthood) are not those that maintain the developed habit.

But confirmed cigarette smoking is by far the most frequent form of tobacco use – and also the most closely associated with disease. An obvious starting point is the question: do cigarette smokers smoke primarily for nicotine? There is strong evidence to show that most do. First, most smokers avoid cigarettes that are low in nicotine. Eighty percent of the cigarettes sold in the UK in 1977 had nicotine deliveries of 1.2 milligrams or more – despite the availability of mild cigarettes which deliver as little as 0.3 mg nicotine and the fact that smokers have been encouraged for five years to switch for health reasons to low-nicotine, low-tar brands.

Second, 80–90% of cigarette smokers inhale. Inhalation makes sense only as a method of nicotine self-administration. The enjoyment of tobacco through smell and taste, and the oral and manipulative satisfactions of smoking, can be obtained without drawing smoke into the lungs.

The third piece of evidence for the importance of nicotine is simply that measuring its level in blood and urine shows that smokers habitually absorb doses large enough to have major pharmacological effects.

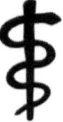

Cigars and Sigmund

World Medicine May 1980

Freud may have been a tobacco addict, but do his theories help us understand the nature of such addiction?

Few aspects of human behaviour avoided Freud's attention, and smoking was no exception. The habit is rich in levels of potential meaning – the phallic shape of the cigar or cigarette, the oral nature of the behaviour and its affinity with taking milk from the breast, and the symbolism of fire.

Yet Freud's involvement with tobacco is interesting as much for the stubborn strength of his own addiction as for any theoretical contribution. He was in many ways a classic casualty. Yet through forty years of suffering from an intermittent but severe "affection of the heart", and through thirty-three operations for a cancer of the oral cavity (which eventually proved fatal) Freud persisted in smoking. His doctors implicated nicotine and strongly recommended abstinence, but without result.

Ernest Jones, Freud's biographer, wrote: "He was always a heavy smoker – twenty cigars a day were his usual allowance

– and he tolerated abstinence from it with the greatest difficulty." During one brief but miserable attempt to give up, Freud himself commented, "renouncing the sweet habit of smoking has resulted in a great diminution of my intellectual interests". The desire to continue to work at maximum capacity was an integral part of his "need" for tobacco. Earlier, when Freud had been confronted by one of his doctors with the clear choice of continuing to smoke at great risk to his heart, or of forsaking the habit, Freud had replied: "I am not following your interdict from smoking; do you think then it is so very lucky to have a long miserable life?" When Freud's pathologist accused nicotine of causing the "leucoplastic growth" (in fact clearly cancerous) which had recently been removed from his mouth, Freud is said merely to have shrugged his shoulders.

Yet Freud's character was not particularly susceptible to addiction. He had been one of cocaine's earliest enthusiasts, advocating its use in a variety of clinical contexts (including anaesthesia), distributing it liberally among family and friends, and himself taking regular doses for depression and indigestion. Though several colleagues became addicted, Freud suffered no ill-effects and believed that any danger in the use of cocaine would come from the newly developed hypodermic needle, not from the drug itself.

There is no evidence that Freud considered the origins of his own addiction, but he incorporated the motivation to smoke in his general theory of sexuality. He argued that thumb-sucking was a re-experiencing of the pleasures of suckling. It was also a source of desirable sensations, and as such could be seen as an "auto-erotic" manifestation of primitive sexuality. Among children who had a "constitutional intensification of the erotogenic significance of the labial region", thumb-sucking would be natural childhood behaviour. As adults, such people would be "epicures in kissing" and would have a powerful motive for smoking and drinking.

In 1946, Edmund Bergler, in *Psychopathology of Compulsive Smoking*, wrote of the habit's childhood antecedents: "Getting something orally is the first great libidinous experience of life: breast, milk bottle, pacifier, food. The smoker reassures himself by getting something into his mouth too." In general, smoking was an "excellent outlet", he said. A. A. Brill, a president of the American Psychoanalytic Association, wrote in the *International Journal of Psychoanalysis* in 1992: "I have never seen a single neurosis or psychosis which could definitely be attributed... to tobacco. On the other hand one is more justified in looking with suspicion at the abstainer... most of the fanatic opponents of tobacco I have known were all bad neurotics." Freud would no doubt have approved.

Nevertheless, psychoanalysts recognised that some smoking could have its origins in a personality disorder. Smoking has been seen as, for example, a substitute for masturbation or a manifestation of masochism (continued smoking in the face of a health risk may be part of an unconscious wish for self-injury). Bergler, writing in the *International Journal of Sexology* in 1953, gave an account of pathological smoking which demonstrated the kind of convoluted logic peculiar to such interpretations. Having suggested that a moderate use of tobacco (along with kissing and "gourmanderie") are aspects of oral eroticism, he subsequently argued that people smoke compulsively not for pleasure, but "as the unconscious defence against the inner reproach of wanting to be refused".

While the psychoanalytic interpretations of compulsive

smoking approach the wilder flights of fancy, the explanation of moderate smoking in terms of orality is at least plausible. W.H. Auden, for example, is said to have explained his heavy smoking as "insufficient weaning – I must have something to suck".

In psychoanalytic literature, it is rare to find hypotheses which are general and unambiguous enough to be tested. But Freudian ideas that smoking has its origins in childhood can – and have been – measured against conventional scientific yardsticks. Is there, then, any evidence that smoking is a feature of an "oral personality"? Do smokers differ from non-smokers in the degree to which they experienced "oral frustration" as children?

In fact there *is* some evidence that the ability to give up smoking has some relation to age at weaning. In a 1958 study conducted by McArthur at Harvard University, light smokers able to stop were found to have spent on average 8 months at their mothers' breast and heavy smokers able to stop 6.8 months, while those who had never tried to give up were weaned at an average age of 5 months, and those who had tried and failed at 4.7 months.

Another link with childhood was found in a 1972 survey by Zucker and Van Horn which looked at the smoking and drinking of men in late adolescence. First-born boys who had been closely followed by a brother or sister tended to smoke more – and to have more drinking problems. This could be because such children would have received less maternal attention during feeding (a narrow interpretation of oral frustration), or (on a broader Freudian view) because most maternal deprivation occurred during the oral phase of development.

Surveys have provided limited evidence for the view that adult smoking may be related to childhood experience. However, there is only slight evidence that smoking is part of a wider "oral personality". In 1979, Howe and Summerfield, two psychologists from Birkbeck College, reported a study which had looked at whether smokers and non-smokers differed in "orality" – as measured by sucking pencils, sweets or a thumb, chewing food or biting nails. There were no significant differences between smokers and non-smokers. There was some evidence of greater orality among smokers who had never succeeded in giving up for any significant time, but even here the differences were in pencil-sucking and nail-biting, but not in thumb-sucking and sweet-eating.

More firmly based is the idea that smoking might be related to other oral behaviours, like drinking alcohol and coffee, which are non-nutritive. Various studies have consistently demonstrated this: in a study of American university students reported by Matarazzo and Saslow, non-smokers drank on average between one and one and a half cups of coffee a day, while smokers drank on average double this amount. In another study, cigarette consumption correlated highly with alcohol intake and with drinking problems.

However, the fact that tobacco, coffee and alcohol tend to be used by the same people can be explained without reference to a concept such as orality. All three substances tend to be consumed in a social context which might attract particular kinds of people. It's also possible that the mood-altering substances of nicotine, caffeine and alcohol may be more useful to those with difficulties in the self-regulation of affect, irrespective of early experience or of any constitutionally intensified "erotogenic significance of the labial region".

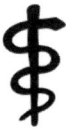

It's not a patch on sucking

The Independent March 1994

If smokers need something to suck, as well as nicotine, a substitute cigarette containing nicotine but little else may be the answer.

The current route for smokers wishing to give up – nicotine gum or patches plus standard anti-smoking advice and encouragement – is proving disappointing. Only one in five smokers wanting to give up is still not smoking a year after the start of their treatment, according to an overview of research published last January in the *Lancet*.

Dr Godfrey Fowler, author of the report, and head of the Department of General Practice at Oxford University, says it is important to remember that without any help at all, only around 1 per cent of those smokers would have given up. "Nevertheless, even in achieving 20 per cent abstinence, the effect of current nicotine replacement therapies is relatively small."

One reason for this is that there is more to smoking than nicotine. Having something distracting to do with the hands and mouth, especially at times of stress, is clearly part of the habit. "As an ex-smoker, I am myself aware that the business of handling cigarettes is important," comments Dr Fowler.

"People who have given up for years are still playing with paperclips and sucking pencils."

To meet the oral needs of smokers will require the development of some form of artificial cigarette which provides both a nicotine fix and an opportunity for ritualised hand-to-mouth behaviour.

"Not the misery of abstinence, with nothing lit between my lips"

The recent emphasis on nicotine addiction has tended to sideline other elements in the tobacco habit. But a century ago, Sigmund Freud was well aware of the complex attractions of smoking. Considering the origins of his own compulsive smoking, he argued that stimulation of the lips was central to the habit's satisfaction.

At the Institute of Psychiatry's Health Behaviour Unit in London, Professor Michael Russell has spent 20 years researching ways to help smokers to quit. "Though the weight of evidence is that people smoke basically because of nicotine, other aspects of the habit are important," he says. "I believe sensory factors become rewarding primarily because they are associated with intake of nicotine. But there is certainly a biological predisposition to conditioning behaviours that involve the hand and mouth."

With this in mind, Professor Russell strongly advocates the development of an alternative to smoking that provides nicotine and that feels like a cigarette. To reduce smoking's toll of death and disability, such a device would have to produce negligible amounts of tar (which leads to lung cancer) and substantially less carbon monoxide (which contributes to

It's not a patch on sucking

heart disease), and ideally none of the noxious gases responsible for chronic bronchitis.

In the eighties, the US tobacco company R J Reynolds spent $300 million developing an artificial cigarette. Professor Russell thinks it came close to producing a device that would save thousands of lives. In the prototype, lighting a carbon ring heated a metal core around which tobacco was wrapped. Instead of being burnt, the heated tobacco gave off a smoke that consisted mostly of water vapour and droplets of the harmless oily liquid glycerine. The smoke contained nicotine, but only 10 per cent of the tar delivered by a conventional cigarette, and some carbon monoxide.

"There were drawbacks," says Professor Russell. "Market testing showed the flavour needed to be improved, the amount of nicotine delivered doubled and the amount of carbon monoxide cut. But then such a device would very likely persuade people to switch from ordinary cigarettes."

Unfortunately, research on artificial cigarettes has stalled. In the US, a House of Representatives sub-committee labelled the Reynolds product a nicotine delivery system, meaning it could not be marketed as a cigarette but would have to be treated as a drug subject to strict controls.

"That was a knee-jerk response: bureaucratic technicalities abetted by misguided pressure from health experts," says Professor Russell. "The climate will improve when people understand there is no good evidence that nicotine itself is harmful at smoking doses, especially when absorbed relatively slowly. Swedish people who smear ground tobacco inside their mouths absorb as much nicotine as cigarette smokers but suffer no more heart and blood vessel disease than those who use no form of tobacco."

If nicotine does not cause harm, there is no rational objection to providing it in a form that smokers find satisfactory, as long as the nicotine is not accompanied by the other elements in smoke that cause disease. Yet tobacco companies in general have paid little attention to purifying the drug they purvey – an attitude that could prove very short-sighted.

The technology for delivering nicotine virtually free from harmful tars and gases requires some further refinement, and the resistance of regulatory authorities must be overcome. But designing a truly less hazardous form of cigarette that provides both the drug and the sensory stimulation smokers need is the logical way forward for those who find themselves genuinely unable to forsake tobacco.

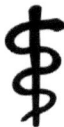

Smoke signals

The Guardian October 1983

The war against smoking is getting nowhere. Is there a snuff solution?

Smoking puzzled Columbus. It puzzles non-smokers still. Why do people so like a particular leaf that they smoke it day in, day out? The habit itself, and what we know about brain chemistry, suggests that the key must be nicotine. First, smokers avoid cigarettes which yield little. "Mild" cigarettes, available and encouraged for ten years, still account for only one in ten smoked.

Secondly, cigarettes mean inhalation. This makes sense only when you remember inhalation is a uniquely effective way of getting a drug to the brain. Neither the ethologists' ideas of displacement activity nor Freud's oral eroticism account for it.

Once in the brain, nicotine has important effects since it mimics the chemical messenger acetylcholine. The molecular structure of the two substances makes nicotine a skeleton key, activating the natural neurotransmitter's receptors in the nervous system.

Once it has produced an acetylcholine response, the nicotine does not disappear as rapidly as the normal chemical. Instead, it stays on, blocking the receptor. Depending on the size and frequency of dose, the effect of nicotine can therefore switch from stimulation to depression. It is a balance over which the smoker has literally fingertip control and probably accounts for the alerting and sedative effects smokers describe. Electrical activity in the brain is evidence for the reality of these apparently contradictory effects.

But nicotine's widespread influence on brain biochemistry also confers addictive potential. Neural mechanisms act to counter its effects so that when the drug is suddenly removed there is the "rebound" experienced as the discomfort of drug withdrawal. Smoking another cigarette instantly restores the artificial balance, and the insidious cycle is perpetuated.

The discovery ten years ago that opiate-like chemicals occur naturally in the brain made sense of thousands of years' use and abuse of an obscure Himalayan poppy. The connection between acetylcholine and nicotine is equally important.

In a sense nicotine is the scourge, since without it people would not smoke. On the other hand, it is probably not the nicotine which is doing us the most harm. There may be a role in heart disease, but it is the carcinogenic tars and irritant gases in cigarette smoke which have the most dramatic effects.

It would help greatly if we devised ways of giving people nicotine they want (because their bodies are chained to it or because they find the drug a tool to manipulate a psychological state) but without exposing them to smoke.

The latest suggestion is "liquid snuff," nicotine solution and cellulose squeezed into the nose. Researchers from the London-based Institute of Psychiatry report in the *British Medical Journal* that "nasal nicotine" leads to effective absorption of the drug, with enough reaching the brain to give a "buzz". Liquid snuff could help smokers quit. But inhalation will take a lot of beating. Around 90 percent of the nicotine present in inhaled smoke reaches the brain in less than seven seconds.

Absorption of nicotine from swallowed tobacco is slow, and much is broken down in the liver before it reaches the brain. Chewing tobacco is possible, but absorption through the membranes of the mouth is also relatively ineffective. Snuffing finely-chopped tobacco is faster: the newly contrived liquid preparations probably speedier still. But even nasal nicotine will not replace the "hit" which a smoker gets in the few seconds following each inhalation of smoke.

Still we are not stuck with smoke forever. We could replace cigarettes with a device delivering metered nicotine as an aerosol spray. The dispenser would be put into the mouth and the vapour drawn into the lungs – as with anti-asthma drugs.

Smoke signals

Absorption of nicotine, and its passage to the brain, would then be just as fast and effective as with inhaled smoke.

Developing new ways of administering nicotine has been under-funded and under-researched. The tobacco industry's interests in diversification might have stretched that far, but they seem to have been surprisingly inactive. One reason given, paradoxically, is that nicotine is too dangerous a substance to dabble with.

Another is that effort has been put into the attempt to make cigarettes themselves less appallingly lethal. Much play has been made of the "wisdom" of taking the low-tar road. Unfortunately the low road is also very likely to lead to a premature dead-end.

The inhaler looks like a good long-term bet. Preliminary research in the States confirms that some smokers find "vaping" an acceptable alternative. But success depends on an increased understanding of the way small particles behave when they are inhaled. This is an area in which tobacco companies' research departments are now active, through commercial constraints may delay dissemination and use of their findings.

Chapter Fifteen

QALYs become the metric of medicine

Are half a dozen hip replacements a better buy than one heart transplant? It depends on quality as well as quantity of life.

The Guardian February 1985

Even when the time-and-motion men have finished with the NHS and we know the cost of every stitch and pill, we will still know the value of very little – until we have agreed ways of assessing health not just as survival but also as quality of life.

Freedom from pain and disability are clearly ingredients in many individual decisions about treatment. People sometimes trade the chance of longer survival for a life that is shorter but not marred by the disfiguring or debilitating effects of surgery or drugs. And there is no shortage of opinion on whether hip replacements that prevent chronic discomfort should have preference over life-saving heart transplants. But can such individual preferences be expressed in a way that allows the value of alternative treatments to be rationally assessed?

Health economists now think they can. The fact that quality of life is inevitably subjective does not mean that it is unmeasurable. The key is a "unit" of health called a

QALYs become the metric of medicine

Quality-Adjusted Life Year (QALY) that combines extension of life with a measure of its worth. And the people who judge how much life is worth are ourselves.

The starting point is a group of individuals — ideally a random sample drawn from the general population — who are asked to imagine different states of pain and disability and rank them from most to least acceptable. People are allowed to say that some states are worse than death. Being in severe pain and bedridden for the rest of your life might be one of them.

The individuals in the sample then assign numbers to these different conditions to indicate how *much* worse one state is than another. This is done on a scale from 0 to 1, with 0 representing death and 1 perfect health. Being chair-bound and in pain might be rated as 0.3, for example; being house-bound but in no pain 0.8. These judgments are averaged to give the value people in general place on living with different degrees of discomfort and disability.

The cost-effectiveness of specific medical interventions can then be calculated. If an operation is certain to move a patient from a state of chair-bound pain to pain-free but limited mobility, it will increase quality of life by 0.5 in our example. If it also extends life by two years, one QALY is gained.

In practice of course it is more complicated. We have to account for the chances of death during surgery, the possibility that the operation will fail to produce the expected gains, and the benefits of alternative treatments. But the principle is plain. The QALY is an all-embracing measure; and it is standard. Like can be compared with like. And the cost in NHS resources of obtaining one QALY can be calculated for any number of different procedures.

A foreign correspondent in medicine

Alan Williams, of York University's department of health economics, presented the QALY concept at a recent meeting on open-heart surgery to bypass partially obstructed coronary arteries. By reducing the risk of a heart attack, coronary artery bypass grafting improves life expectancy for some patients. For others crippled by angina, its benefit lies more in reduction of discomfort and disability. So a measure that combines survival with quality of life is especially appropriate.

The QALYs Professor Williams applied to coronary artery operations were based on health evaluations made by a panel of seventy people. Using their assessments, he was able to say that in patients with critical coronary disease, bypass surgery produced a QALY at a cost of £800. But in patients with less serious disease, the cost per QALY was over £3000.

"This method does not tell you what a QALY itself is worth. I don't know whether we should be spending £500 to get one QALY or £5000," says Alan Williams. "All I can say is that you'll get more QALYs if you put your money into one procedure rather than another. But that is some sort of breakthrough." For comparison, he calculated that the price for one QALY through heart transplantation is indeed £5000. For a kidney transplant it is £3000; and for replacing a hip £750.

For most of those at the meeting, the QALY was a novel idea. But there was consensus that however fast Nigel Lawson mints pounds, doctors will find ways of spending them; and setting priorities is therefore inevitable. To some extent, the problem is compounded by the public's double standards. On the one hand we accept that life at any price makes neither economic nor ethical sense. On the other, outrage at an individual "being left to die" is easily kindled.

QALYs provide a kind of answer. In Alan Williams' terms,

"They reflect the calmer decisions people make about resource allocation when their emotions are not directly engaged."

One objection to their use is that QALYs put an economist's calculator in the place of a caring relationship. But health economists reply that they are reflecting not their own judgments but ours. A rational approach to medical priorities is better, they say, than the present position in which the NHS is tugged this way and that by competing appeals, and where most resources go to those who pluck the heartstrings hardest.

Postscript

At Alan Williams' talk [in 1984], not everyone was impressed with the new beast on the block. "The QALY. What kind of economic animal is that?" was one disparaging comment. "One with a lot of growth potential and a very long life expectancy" might have been the answer. Alan Williams' paper on the health economics of coronary artery bypass grafting, published in August 1985, came to be recognised as one of the most influential ever written in its field.

The QALY, with refinements, became the standard way for organisations such as NICE to evaluate new treatments and determine whether they were worth funding. The flip side of a QALY – the Disability-Adjusted Life Year, or DALY – became the standard way of measuring and ranking the global impact of chronic diseases from depression to diabetes.

Alan Williams died of cancer at the age of 77. His *Guardian* obituary records that he had always been an advocate of the idea of a "fair innings" when it comes to life expectancy. Someone who dies at 25 has been cheated of that, while someone who dies after the traditional three score years and ten has not. So, once his own prognosis became clear, he said he could hardly complain – though he regretted leaving so much undone.

Chapter Sixteen

Communication key to better care

VIDEOPHONE OFFERS LONG-DISTANCE DIAGNOSIS

Electronic wizardry may soon allow specialists to examine patients who are hundreds of miles away.

The Independent September 1993

Your child has a sore throat. You have a home videophone, which simultaneously transmits voice and high quality pictures. You ask your child to open wide and say "aaah". You thrust the camcorder at his throat. In the surgery, the doctor looks at the screen and tells you whether your child needs to be brought in for a face-to-face consultation.

Shopping and banking from home are now possible. In the not-too-distant future, electronic wizardry could bring healthcare into our homes as well. For the moment, we are not likely to see GPs' crowded waiting rooms replaced by TV screens. But family doctors are experimenting with "telemedicine" as a means of obtaining specialist clinical opinion.

Most interest in the idea has come from remote rural areas. By the end of the year [1993], Dr John Wynn-Jones hopes to be video-linking patients from the small town of Montgomery, in mid-Wales, with hospital consultants many

Videophone offers long-distance diagnosis

miles away. This will be the first telemedicine project in the UK.

Among the pioneers are doctors in the Norwegian city of Tromso which lies above the Arctic Circle and is far from Oslo, where most specialist medicine is practiced. In February, the Tromso University Hospital established a department of telemedicine, which offers more than half a million people living in remote communities a service that ranges from psychiatry to the interpretation of X-rays. One specialist area is the long-distance diagnosis of skin complaints.

During a videoconference, the patient explains the problem to the consultant, and this account is supplemented by the GP. "Then the camera is focused on the area of skin in question and transmits either a live image or a higher-quality still picture," explains Gjermund Hartviksen, a computer scientist at the Tromso department. An initial trial involving two hundred new dermatology cases showed complete agreement between diagnosis at a distance and by a visit from the local specialist.

The Norwegian experience suggests that remote diagnosis is equally effective for ear, nose and throat complaints, which can be examined with special miniature cameras. Two-way videolinks are also providing a treatment service in adolescent psychiatry. "It works well. The young people are relaxed in front of a camera, and sometimes more at ease than when they meet the doctor face to face," Dr Hartviksen says.

In Montgomery, Dr Wynn-Jones is keen to explore telemedicine as a tool in radiology. "At the moment, I can wait up to a week for a specialist opinion on an X-ray," he says. "The delay is frustrating for me and an anxious one for the patient."

Hospitals in mid-Wales still use conventional X-ray film.

But the Hammersmith Hospital in west London has developed a system in which X-ray images are stored digitally on discs. This combines compact storage, easy access and, crucially, the ability to transfer images by phone. If the Hammersmith can prove the technology works, we could have radiologists from all over the country reporting on X-rays, says Dr Wynn-Jones.

A pilot study in Staffordshire has shown that ECGs can be sent en route to hospital for expert analysis after heart attacks. A nurse riding with the ambulance recorded ECGs from patients and transmitted the electronic data by cell phone. At the hospital, staff diagnosed cases where the cause of chest pain was definitely cardiac. These patients were admitted to a prepared bed, saving an hour's wait in A&E.

In the archives of Dr Wynn-Jones' practice is a photograph of a former partner returning from a home visit with a kidney bowl in one hand and a pheasant in the other. In the future, he may well be carrying a 12-lead ECG and portable computer videophone.

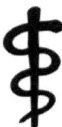

Breaking down the barriers

World Medicine July 1982

Why do doctors and patients so often confuse one another?

I told a friend I was writing an article on doctor-patient communication. "That'll be easy," she said. "There isn't any."

That view was base on her individual experiences as a patient. I was surprised to find an equally critical account from Lorraine Sherr, a psychologist at the University of Warwick, who has made a systematic study of patients' reactions to routine antenatal screening. Her conclusion is that the women didn't know why they were there; the doctors didn't know that the women didn't know; the women were too afraid to ask; and the doctors were too bored to tell them.

David Pendleton is the first non-medically qualified researcher to receive a Fellowship from the Royal College of General Practitioners. Dr Pendleton's brief is to travel the country encouraging GPs to look critically at the way they work. "GPs would like to look at their consultations but at the moment are not sure what to look *for*," he says. Aided by videotapes, David Pendleton thinks he is now able to show them both the extent of the problem and what can be done about it.

In an early study, Dr Pendleton and colleagues from the Oxford University Department of Psychology asked GPs to fill in a questionnaire after a total of 920 consultations. One question asked if there had been any problems in communication. In almost a quarter of cases, there had been. Sometimes the difficulty was that the patient seemed not to have been convinced by the advice or information given. Generally this was seen as stemming from lack of trust in the doctor and not from any failure to understand. But far more common were problems in communicating in the other direction, from patient to doctor. Sometimes the patient was thought to have deliberately withheld information.

A foreign correspondent in medicine

Patients of course have a rather different view. A study asked them to think of a consultation which had been particularly good, and one which had been particularly bad, and give reasons. Consultations judged good had been quick, thorough, and led to effective treatment. But only a third of patients' comments were about that task-related side of the proceedings. Two thirds centred on social and emotional factors.

Most frequently expressed was the desire that doctors should take the patients seriously, show concern and give them confidence. Being offered reassurance and having effective treatment were independent causes of the patient feeling satisfied with the consultation.

Chapter Seventeen

Taking drugs and alcohol on board

THE REAL INSIDE STORY

Drug smugglers go to extraordinary lengths to bring heroin and cocaine into the country. Customs officers, aided by doctors, resort to equally extraordinary techniques to catch them.

The Independent September 1992

Last week a woman died in hospital after packages of drugs, thought to be cocaine, burst inside her, causing a massive overdose. Clara Ayemenre, a Nigerian, collapsed at Heathrow's Terminal 3 before reaching customs. Surgeons at Ashford Hospital in west London who operated on her found 84 packages in her stomach.

Other couriers are luckier. Although being caught means they face punishment, medical techniques usually mean their contraband is discovered and removed before it kills them.

Customs officers have the power to detain, for an initial period of 96 hours, anyone they suspect of carrying drugs internally. Of all the messy jobs in the world, taking suspected drug "swallowers" to the lavatory and then sifting through their faeces to find small packets of swallowed heroin and cocaine must be one of the least appealing. But it is a daily task for the customs and medical officers who work in the custody suites at Heathrow.

In the days of the Portaloo and the plastic bag, the work was really unsavoury; it involved a spatula, colander and perfumed face mask. Now the "throne room" is all stainless steel, perspex and transparent plumbing. The washing down of drug packages takes place in a sealed sluice, from which only the contraband emerges to be submitted for analysis.

The number of swallowed drug packages recovered is usually between 80 and 150. The drugs are wrapped in condoms, balloons or cling-film, forming neat packages about the size of a large grape, and swallowed with syrup to make them more palatable. Couriers take a constipating agent before they embark and tend not to eat during the flight.

"Stuffers" use any orifice available

Apart from the damage their trade does to the health of others, smugglers who use their bodies as a vehicle for drugs put their own lives on the line. If a package of heroin comes open in transit, the chance of death is high. When a detainee passes an empty condom, he is rushed to hospital. It may just be the outer wrapping of several layers, but it may equally well be the first sign of a medical emergency.

Another risk is intestinal obstruction caused by packets jamming together in the gut, so any sign of abdominal pain must be taken very seriously. Laxatives are unwise in this situation, since increasing the fluid content of the faeces could lead packages to swell and burst. The surgical removal of swallowed drugs from detainees at Heathrow is required two or three times a year, and hospitals in Uxbridge and Ashford are well acquainted with the problem.

"Stuffers", as opposed to "swallowers", will use any orifice available. The vagina in particular proves commodious, especially in women who have had several children; a photograph in one case record shows a package the dimensions of a decent-sized marrow that was carried into the country this way.

Having stopped a passenger on suspicion, customs officers must look for evidence. A strip search – which detainees can refuse until their appeal is heard by either a senior customs officer or a magistrate – will only reveal what is visible on the naked body. And while grease around the anus or a protruding string clearly give the game away, the suspect can still refuse an intimate body search.

If the detainee does agree to a medical examination of body orifices, the fingers of the examining doctor may be able to detect vaginal packages, or those concealed in the rectum. One of Heathrow Customs' two medical assistants has earned the nickname "Goldfinger" because of his expertise.

An unusual case of pot belly

When it comes to the "swallowers", X-rays provide useful information: packages in the gastrointestinal tract show up because of air trapped within the wrapping. The British Medical Journal once published a paper describing this technique of detection under the title *An Unusual Case of Pot Belly*. But women typically plead pregnancy as a means of avoiding X-rays, and men are also within their rights in refusing to submit to this examination.

All swallowed packages leak, however tightly they are tied, and the drug is absorbed into the bloodstream to be excreted by the kidneys. One of the most useful medical tools of the investigators' trade is a sophisticated laboratory device that detects trace quantities of drugs in urine.

Some passengers test positive because of drugs they have taken for legitimate medical reasons, and they must be carefully excluded. Others may have taken illegal drugs, but before embarkation, and that cannot be held against them. But a drug level in urine that increases over the hours after arrival is good evidence that packages are concealed internally. Such evidence is sufficient for suspects to be taken before magistrates and remanded back into Customs' custody for an extended period of detention.

If all possible searches have failed or been refused, it is a waiting game, as one medical officer recalls: "A suspect was remanded on the evidence of a positive urine test and my statement saying I had felt three packages in the rectum. But over the next 48 hours the detainee refused to eat or drink, and nothing was passed. At the second court attendance, the magistrate said he had no case to answer and he was released. But shortly afterwards Customs re-arrested the man. Over the next day, he passed 37 drug packages."

The longest time officers have waited for a suspect to deliver is 19 days, a performance that would put the most anal retentive personality to shame.

A question Customs officers are always asked is how they decide whom to stop in the first place. The origin of a flight certainly attracts attention: West Africa, Pakistan and Colombia are obvious sources of drugs. Over a recent six-month period, half of the 149 Heathrow suspects who appeared before Uxbridge magistrates were accused of cocaine smuggling. Almost 10 per cent were Colombians.

Nevertheless, the majority of defendants were British; and for these people, the likelihood of being stopped is often determined as much by the way they leave the country as by how they enter it. A suitcase containing condoms in unusually large quantities excites suspicion. So, too, do large amounts of dental floss, since it is used to tie drug packages. Other suspects are earmarked for detention when they return because of intelligence gathered in this country.

There is said to be a particular way of walking that comes from having a rectum full of drugs, but an officer I spoke to thought that was not a significant factor. Neither did he regard profuse sweating and agitation as a good guide. It certainly cannot be that the traffickers look guilty, since we all do. "I don't like going through customs myself," he said.

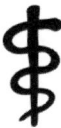

Drunk? But not a drop passed my lips

Can you get intoxicated by inhaling the fumes from other people's booze?

The Independent December 1993

Fed up with passive smoking at parties? Why not try passive drinking instead? It may sound improbable – and do not expect a traffic policeman to believe you – but significant amounts of alcohol can enter the body simply by breathing in the fumes.

I was alerted to this possibility following a publisher's party last Christmas in Oxford. The woman charged with dispensing the simmering punch for the entire evening touched not a drop of her own concoction. Honestly, officer. But she felt distinctly odd by the end of the party, and woke next morning with a hell of a hangover.

A chance discussion with an American while flying from Chicago to London roused my interest further. This man said distillery workers are convinced that inhalation is one route to intoxication. He had spent a year in Lynchburg, Tennessee, working for Jack Daniels. "We were high every night after the shift," he said, "even in the bottling plant where there were huge extractors to take away the fumes."

Cooks are familiar with the idea that alcohol evaporates from a pot during heating. It simply disappears into thin air. For this reason, too much coq au vin, though a perfect description of inebriated impropriety, has never been a convincing excuse for it.

Those with illicit stills in outhouses know perfectly well that the products of heated homemade wine can be collected and condensed, with the appropriate apparatus. So why shouldn't alcohol vapour that is breathed condense in the lungs?

A Bible in the matter of drugs, *Gaddum's Pharmacology* (written by Sir John Gaddum in 1940 and updated ever since) is clear that inhalation is an option for taking alcohol on board. After noting rather prissily that alcohol is an anaesthetic, a disinfectant and an irritant, Gaddum admits that in "discreet doses" it can also be regarded as a valuable tranquilliser, absorbed either from the stomach or as vapour through the lungs.

Dr Peter Taberner, senior lecturer in the Department of Pharmacology at the University of Bristol, has worked on methods of measuring alcohol levels in the body. One of these was to analyse the alcohol content of fluid that bathes the eye. This option, involving the use of an eye patch, was intended for people brought to hospital too drunk to co-operate with a breath test or blood sample. Dr Taberner thinks that one would have to work rather hard to inhale enough alcohol to become intoxicated. But it could be done.

"Glue contains organic solvents similar to ethanol, and clearly they can be inhaled. You can also certainly get an immediate buzz from inhaling alcohol fumes," he says. "If you heated alcohol and had a towel over your head, as if you were taking a cold cure, it would be possible to breathe in enough to have a more prolonged effect. But alcohol vapour is an unpleasant irritant to the lungs; drinking it is far easier."

A Scandinavian friend once told me why the interest in saunas is not completely accounted for by the pleasures of plunging superheated bodies into an ice-cold lake. Nordic folk know that alcoholic spirit poured on to smouldering birch twigs can be breathed in to good effect. It takes merely seconds for the desired substance to go from lungs to blood to brain compared to 20 minutes or so when sluggish absorption of the stomach is relied upon.

Inhalation of alcohol fumes has been tried in the laboratory. Researchers managed to raise blood alcohol levels to 10mg per 100ml in tests on volunteers carried out in

Germany in the fifties and in Britain in 1975. That is a significant amount, although well below the legal limit.

But more popular than alcohol inhalation for intoxication has been the practice of sniffing ether. In the last century, both the drinking and inhalation of ether were widespread in central Europe and in Ulster. Ether abuse was introduced to Northern Ireland by an alcoholic physician in Draperstown who had "taken the pledge" but found in ether an equally effective intoxicant that bypassed the small print. Others followed his example.

So could inhalation of alcohol itself ever become a popular route to intoxication? I doubt it, but it gives a new slant to the idea of a "quick snifter".

Chapter Eighteen

Speculations in obstetrics

THE ULTIMATE TEST TUBE BABY

Aldous Huxley predicted it would be six centuries before babies could be "grown" outside a woman's womb. But this aspect of his brave new world is already more fact that fiction.

The Sunday Telegraph November 1997

This is the Central London Hatchery for humans in the Year of Ford 632. Eggs in surgically removed ovaries are ripened, fertilised with sperm on the lab bench, cloned and connected to an artificial circulation, lung and waste filter for their nine months' gestation. When fully formed, the bottled babies are ready not for birth but for decanting into a nursery where social conditioning completes the process that biological engineering has begun – the creation of human slaves happy in their servitude.

Huxley wrote *Brave New World* in 1932. Little more than sixty years later, two of the four developments needed for the Hatchery's breeding programme – in vitro fertilisation and cloning – are already in place. A third, the maturation of eggs in excised ovaries, will be possible within 5–10 years, while the artificial womb is more fact that fiction. So how far off is a baby, conceived and grown in the lab?

Since the birth of Louise Brown, the world's first "test tube baby", in 1978, more than 150,000 children have begun life in the laboratory. Earlier this year [1997], Dolly the sheep became the first cloned mammal. Only ethics constrain the application of the same technology to humans. Meanwhile, the ripening of mature eggs from frozen slices of ovary will be routine within the decade, according to Professor Robert Winston, director of Britain's largest in vitro fertilisation clinic, at the Hammersmith Hospital.

Scientists are tackling the fourth element in Huxley's vision – the artificial womb – from both the beginning and the end of intrauterine life. They now have the ability to keep embryos alive for half the 14-day period allowed under then 1990 Human Fertilisation and Embryology Act. The embryos are cultured in nutrient fluids, which mimic natural womb secretions, in the week between fertilisation and implantation.

At the other end of pre-birth development, advances in neonatal care mean that premature babies of only 24 weeks' gestation can be supported in hospital incubators through the four months they should still be in the womb. Before 24 weeks, the foetal lungs are still too immature to oxygenate blood, and this is limiting the further development of care based in incubators.

It is the fate of these very premature babies – delivered before 24 weeks and almost certain to die – that is motivating researchers in Tokyo, who have developed the most advanced artificial womb so far. In July, Yoshinori Kuwabara, professor of obstetrics at Juntendo University, and colleagues announced that they had removed a 17-week-old goat foetus from its mother and placed it in an acrylic tank filled with simulated amniotic fluid. The foetus was supplied with nutrient-enriched and oxygenated blood until the time came for it to be "born" three weeks later.

Professor Kuwabara estimates that the stage at which the goat was removed from its mother corresponds to a human gestation of 20 weeks. "Maybe within 10 years we will have made the move from animals to humans," he says.

Roger Gosden, professor of reproductive biology at Leeds University, is one of many British doctors who believe that such research is ethically justified. "Take as an example a woman who develops a life-threatening cancer while carrying a dearly wanted pregnancy," he speculates. "Treatment to save the mother will kill the foetus. But you could conceivably take out the woman's womb with the baby still in it and connect up the blood vessels serving the placenta to some form of life-support system. Or you could remove the foetus and try to link blood vessels in the baby's umbilical cord to the same sort of equipment."

Cardiopulmonary bypass machines developed to take over the circulation during open heart surgery are highly effective, kidney dialysis is well advanced, and drugs now limit damage to the blood caused by contact with the artificial surfaces of tubes and other equipment.

This scenario, of long-term life support to a foetus which would otherwise die, is also acceptable to the Society for the Protection of Unborn Children. "If the artificial womb is used to save the life of very premature babies, there would be no problem," says Brendan Gerard.

There are, however, technical difficuties to overcome:

success requires not just an artificial womb but an artificial placenta too. This immensely sophisticated organ allows oxygen and nutrients to pass in one direction while waste products flow in the other. It also acts as a highly selective filter of maternal blood. "The placenta does the job of the foetus' lungs, kidneys, liver and digestive system," says Professor Gosden. "It also allows through maternal antibodies which protect the newborn against infection."

The placenta is supremely adaptable and changes with the needs of the foetus. "The most critical time is between two weeks, when the foetus is still a mass of identical cells, and three months, when you have a recognisably human foetus," according to Dr Rosa Beddington, of the division of mammalian development at the MRC labs in Mill Hill, London. "Cells are becoming specialised and moving around. The embryo is deciding where its head and tail should be. Any deficiency in the delivery of oxygen and nutrients will result in abnormalities and retarded growth."

Producing an artificial placenta is still beyond science. But few would argue it is impossible, and there is certainly a demand on medical grounds. Cases would include women who cannot carry a baby to term because of a danger to their health or repeated miscarriage, or because they were born without a womb or have had a hysterectomy. At the moment, their only answer is surrogacy.

But there is a suspicion that the artificial womb would also prove attractive to women who want a child without the bother of being pregnant. "Using an artificial womb for women capable of having a normal pregnancy is difficult to imagine, but ethical sensibilities change," says Juliet Tizzard, director of Progress Educational Trust, a charity which fosters public understanding of reproductive science. "Carrying the foetus and feeling it move are part of the process of bonding. But successful adoptions show that you don't have to go through pregnancy to bond with a child."

Pro-life groups, on the other hand, see the prospect as an affront to humanity. "We would not countenance the artificial womb in this situation," asserts Brendan Gerard of SPUC. "The woman is the natural custodian of the child up to birth and has the responsibility of safeguarding the embryo with her body."

Postscript

In 2018, a team from Edinburgh was the first to mature human eggs in the laboratory from their most primitive form to a stage when they are capable of being fertilised. Professor Kuwabara died in 2000, but in 2017 researchers in Philadelphia used an artificial sack of amniotic fluid to keep alive lamb foetuses equivalent to a human gestation of 22–23 weeks. The animals were "born" up to four weeks later. As foreseen by Roger Gosden, the lambs' umbilical cords were connected to a device that oxygenated their blood. But researchers said that such an artificial womb would not be able to support a human foetus for a full gestation.

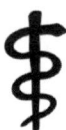

A foreign correspondent in medicine

CAN A FOETUS FEEL PAIN?

Foetal pain is highlighted by anti-abortionists but its implications extend beyond their agenda to the process of birth itself.

The Independent February 1997

Giving a blood transfusion in the womb is the only way of saving the life of an unborn baby with severe anaemia. A doctor pushes the hollow transfusion needle into the mother's abdomen, through the placenta, and straight into a vein in the tiny liver. Ultrasound scans recorded on video show how foetuses respond.

"At least from the age of 20 weeks onwards, they move all over the place, arms and legs waving as they try to get away from the needle," says Professor Nicholas Fisk, of Queen Charlotte's Hospital, London, who has pioneered such life-saving procedures in the womb. Are those foetuses feeling pain, or are they taking only reflex avoiding action?

In the bitter struggle between those who favour a woman's right to choose and those who consider abortion an evil, this question is proving a crucial battleground. A *Panorama* programme, soon to be screened to mark the 30th anniversary of the Abortion Act, is said to make great play of the suffering potentially caused to foetuses by terminations carried out close to the legal limit of 24 weeks.

The issue of foetal pain looks set to be exploited by the "pro-lifers", especially in the run-up to the [1997] election – even though 90 per cent of terminations take place before 13 weeks, when doctors agree it is simply not an issue. But the implications extend well beyond this highly emotive area. If foetuses really can feel pain, then surgeons operating on them in the womb will want to ensure adequate analgesia. And whether the long trauma of birth itself should be accompanied by pain relief for the baby as well as the mother becomes a real question.

During vaginal delivery, each contraction rams the baby's head against the opening in the pelvis until it is squashed into a shape that will pass through. One in 10 babies is born with the additional aid of forceps, or a vacuum sucker to help drag them by the head through the birth canal. "There could be a good argument for this being painful," says Professor Fisk. The same is true of the responses he sees during foetal surgery.

Clearly we cannot ask the foetus what it feels. But Professor Fisk believes that we can understand more about what it is experiencing by measuring how the foetal hormones and brain blood flow react to stimuli that we would find painful.

With a grant from the Wellbeing charity, he is now midway through a programme of research that will shed light on this important area. Small amounts of blood taken from a 20-week foetus at the time the transfusion needle enters the liver show that levels of the stress hormone cortisol double and levels of the body's own pain-relieving opiate chemicals increase six-fold. There is also a highly significant increase in blood flow in the brain.

Despite such evidence of a physical stress response, some doctors are convinced that foetal pain is a complete non-issue. "Foetal pain is a misnomer at any stage of foetal development," Dr Stuart Derbyshire, formerly of Salford's Hope Hospital and now at the University of Pittsburgh, has argued. His certainty is based on the belief that the experience of pain requires not just unpleasant sensations but also emotional and cognitive components that are simply not present in the unborn baby. It is a mistake to say that biological development is enough, he claims.

A quite different view is taken by Dr Vivette Glover, a senior clinical scientist at Queen Charlotte's. "I disagree with the idea that you need any cognitive ability or prior experience to have a simple feeling of pain," she says.

It is accepted that an organism must be conscious to feel pain, and evidence from studies of people who have suffered brain injury suggests that the cortex of the brain must be functioning for anyone to be conscious. So when is the cortex of the foetus all wired up and working?

Around 24 weeks is the earliest age at which premature babies survive. At this stage of development, the cortex is "lit up" in terms of its electrical activity. But because we cannot record from the baby still inside the womb, we do not know whether there is activity in the cortex before this point.

"The earliest time at which a foetus might possibly feel something is 14 weeks," says Dr Glover. "That is when the first nerve fibres from the outside world arrive at the cortex. These are not themselves pain fibres, but in the adult they are involved in the fight or flight response, so they might mediate distress.

"Between then and 24 weeks or so, when all the anatomical pain pathways are in place, is a grey area. But until we know more, and taking the mother's well-being always into account, we should be giving the foetus the benefit of the doubt."

It is startling to recall that as recently as 10 years ago

doctors did not give pain relief to new-born babies undergoing surgery. The assumption was that they did not feel pain. "Now it would be unethical not to give analgesia even to a premature baby of 26 weeks," says Professor Fisk. "When women ask us whether a foetus of the same age having surgery can feel pain, the traditional answer has been 'No'. But we have a duty to find out if this is true."

This is especially so in the light of growing evidence from animal studies that stress experienced as a foetus can affect long-term development of the nervous system and sensitivity to pain. There is no certainty that this is the case with the human foetus. But we do know that one effect of circumcision in the first week of life is to increase response to pain six months later. Research from Montreal shows that immunisation causes a far longer period of crying in boys who have been circumcised than in those who have not.

The Queen Charlotte's team is now trying to discover whether the stress response in foetuses undergoing surgery can be reduced by giving a pain-killing drug such as fentanyl. Even if it were certain that the mature foetus felt pain, doctors could not give analgesia without establishing first that it was effective and secondly that it was safe.

Fentanyl is a narcotic agent. To give it to the mother in concentrations that would cross the placenta risks interfering with the mother's breathing, and whether it is practical and safe to give it to the foetus has still to be proved.

This cautious approach to pain relief during foetal surgery is backed by Peter Hepper, director of the Foetal Behaviour Research Centre at Queen's University, Belfast. But the question of pain relief during a late termination is different. Here there is no question of analgesia doing long-term damage. "In my view," he says, "the person who suffers most from abortion is the woman. And if pain relief for the foetus becomes practical, she should be the one to choose whether or not it is given."

Accepting the reality of foetal pain should not contradict a woman's right to choose, most doctors involved in this area would argue. "But people's attitude towards termination often colours their attitude to the subject of foetal pain in general. This seems wrong," says Dr Glover. "People on both sides of the abortion debate can agree that the aim is to cause as little suffering as possible".

What the foetus does and when

7–8 weeks	Beginnings of spontaneous movement
8–14 weeks	Reflex reaction to touch, starting with the lips and spreading to rest of body
13 weeks	Electrical activity seen in the lowest part of the brain (brainstem)
20–24 weeks	Foetus moves in response to loud noise. Physical stress response to stimuli we feel as pain
24 weeks	Electrical activity in cortex. All anatomical pathways needed to feel pain are in place. Many healthy premature babies survive
37–40 weeks	Full-term birth

Chapter Nineteen

Christmas crackers

DING-DONG MERRILY ON HIGH, FLY BY WITH SANTA'S MUSHROOM

World Medicine December 1981

Santa Claus makes sense only when seen as the relic of a psychedelic mushroom cult practised in the witch-doctoring days of our Northern European ancestors.

If that sounds unlikely, consider the jolly old gentleman a little more closely. Clothed in bright red and white, he hails from some far distant snowy wasteland, flies through the air drawn by a rowdy gang of reindeer, and arrives, bringing gifts, down the chimney. An improbable collection of attributes by any standards – but not, according to Rogan Taylor, an anthropologist at Lancaster University, a random one.

There is good evidence for his unorthodox view of the origins of our cheerful Christmas character. The clues are distant, but not in time. Until recently, the nomadic Siberian tribes retained a religious tradition in which the witch-doctor, or shaman, mediates between the lower and upper spirit worlds and the middle region which humans inhabit like the filling in a cosmic sandwich. In several respects, these shamans resemble Father Christmas.

Like Santa, the shaman brings gifts — although these are of wisdom and healing rather than material possessions. Like Santa, the shaman uses the "chimney", a smoke-hole cut in the roof of the tribesmen's snow-bound yurt dwellings, which is both a practical entrance and symbolic of the return to earth. Third, it is in midwinter that the shaman is most active — because darkness offers evil spirits their greatest opportunity.

For more evidence we must turn from man to mushroom. The relevant fungus is the fly agaric, *Amanita muscaria*, plentiful in the autumn woods of Eurasia, and especially in the northern forests of birch and pine.

Shamans used this mushroom in their healing seances, and sensations of feeling extraordinarily light on the feet, flying, and travelling great distances accompany its euphoriant and hallucinatory effects. It also seems that reindeer have a passion for eating *Amanita* which rivals that of their herdsmen. Hence the mode of travel and merry intoxication of both Santa and his four-legged friends.

But the most striking connection between Santa and the fly agaric is their similar appearance. *Amanita* has a bright red "toadstool" cap, often flecked with white patches remaining from the membrane out of which the mushroom head emerges. Sometimes these remnants look remarkably like a white frill bordering the rich red dome.

Of course there are other elements in our Santa Claus, like the original Saint Nicholas, patron of children (and also of sailors, virgins, and thieves). But as this Christian idea spread it would have naturally assimilated myths indigenous

Ding-dong merrily on high, fly by with Santa's mushroom

to pagan Europe, such as those surrounding shamanistic practices. Interestingly, the myths may now have gone full circle. Arriving back in Siberia, the western European Father Christmas has been taken for a white-bearded old shaman.

One curious practice associated with the shamans and their magic mushroom which has not carried over into our Christmas festivities is that of drinking urine. Siberians who have eaten fly agaric urinate into bowls and then drink the contents to become re-intoxicated, presumably because a proportion of the psychotropic substance in the fungus is excreted unchanged or as an active metabolite. In addition to muscarine and acetylcholine, the amanita contains the hallucinogens muscimol and ibotenic acid.

Perhaps because of this, reindeer also consume human urine and will fight each other for access to pee-holes in the snow. Early western travellers, unaware of this penchant, put themselves at risk – as is recorded by Waldemar Jochelson, who was with the Jesup North Pacific Expedition of 1905. "Reindeer have a keen sense of smell but their sight is poor," he wrote. "A man stopping to urinate in the open attracts reindeer from afar which run to the urine, hardly discerning the man, whose position is rather critical when reindeer are coming down on him at full speed."

Although the habit of drinking urine may have been lost, our language – faithful guide, as ever, to the origins of concepts we now take for granted – has preserved the idea in the expression "getting pissed". The literally translated Siberian equivalent is "bemushroomed".

RG Wasson, retired Wall Street banker and fungophile, who did most to extend knowledge of the fly agaric cult, comes close to advocating a return to the original practice.

He writes: "The fixation of our western world on alcohol, often a stultifying intoxicant and seldom an invigorating one, closes our minds to other inebriants older than our fermented drinks and in their effects utterly different."

It is plausible to suggest that the near-divine virtues of the mushroom might have been actively suppressed by those jealous of its secrets and keen to obscure pagan practices. The fungi themselves are mysterious, even dangerous. There is a close association with decay, or worse – think of the Death Cap, Destroying Angel and Devil's bolete – and something sinister in their overnight arrival, apparently without sowing or seed, as if they had been laid as bait for the unwary. Their appearance is totally unlike that of any other plant, and the frequent suggestion of the phallus brings them under the taboos of both sex and death.

Postscript

The Death And Resurrection Show: From Shaman To Superstar by Rogan Taylor was published in 1985.

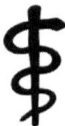

The Christmas edition of the *British Medical Journal* is traditionally one in which not-so-serious topics are considered seriously. The paper on Ambridge's vital statistics (page 144) is one example. Here are two others.

HEALER, DEALER, HEART STEALER: PORTRAYALS OF THE DOCTOR IN POPULAR MUSIC

British Medical Journal Christmas issue December 2014. Nick Surawy Stepney [NSS] was co-author.

Typing "doctor + lyrics" into a well known search engine retrieved 8.4 million results – far more than the 1.3 million hits generated by a similar search involving "lawyer". Doctors are intimately involved in our lives from birth until death, so it is perhaps not surprising that musicians are interested in them.

The portrayal of doctors in popular music is revealing and varied. In *Goodness Gracious Me*, Sophia Loren and Peter Sellers sing of a doctor who has innocently stolen his patient's heart. By contrast, in *One of Us Cannot be Wrong*, Leonard Cohen's doctor has a lustful obsession with the love life of his patient. A New York physician noted for supplying amphetamines is the subject of *Dr Robert* by the Beatles; and The Rolling Stones' *Dear Doctor* concerns a request – made less than a year after the first such transplant – for a surgeon to replace the singer's heart.

In 2012 *The Guardian*'s music blog asked readers to recommend songs about doctors. Although contributors were not representative of the wider population, the list was probably compiled by people unconnected with the medical profession. The blog provided a degree of objectivity and a more manageable volume of material than that generated by an internet search.

A preliminary assessment of the songs in the blog, supplemented by our own knowledge, suggested three themes: the doctor as provider of illicit drugs; other forms of unprofessional conduct, typically sexual involvement with patients; and doctors in their caring role – either literally, or metaphorically as healers of love sickness and broken hearts.

The first 75 songs on the list were categorised by NSS into one of the above themes according to their lyrics, and a random sample of 25 songs was categorised by RS. Songs that did not fit into any of these three themes were classed as "other." Lyrics could not be found for 11 songs, and the meaning of some lyrics was open to a variety of interpretations. A further complication was occasional inconsistencies in the lyrics transcribed on different websites. Even so, our assignment of songs to categories agreed in 80% of cases. Disagreements were resolved by discussion.

Inappropriate behaviour

We expected the theme of doctor as dealer to feature strongly, but this was found in only three of the 64 songs reviewed (5%). This role is implicit in the Beatles' *Dr Robert* and in the Dirty Pretty Things' *Doctors and Dealers* (which describes "crackpot quacks with cracked up egos"), but is perhaps most graphically portrayed in Dr Feelgood's *Down at the Doctors*.

Suggestions of other forms of professional misconduct are more common (19 songs, 30%), including romantic or overtly sexual relationships. In *I'm Your Man*, Leonard Cohen makes several suggestions including "If you want a doctor, I'll examine every inch of you." In the context of the song, this is not an innocent suggestion. The *Doctor of Physick* sung about by Fairport Convention is a clear abuser: "Take care, daughter dear, for the doctor comes to steal your goods in the dead of night ... He'll find young ladies pure as fallen snow; he'll have you all. Doctor Monk unpacks his trunk tonight."

Despite the examples above, it should be noted that most of these inappropriate relationships are initiated by the patient. In *The Physician*, Cole Porter laments that "Of all his sweeties, I had the sweetest diabetes, but he never said he loved me." The doctor "went through wild ecstatics when I showed him my lymphatics" and "did a double hurdle when I shook my pelvic girdle." And yet he refused "to cure that ache in my heart".

Sophia Loren begins with a similar problem in *Goodness Gracious Me*. Although the doctor recounts his expertise in dealing with conditions ranging from beriberi to dysentery, influenza, whooping cough, and night starvation, it is only after extensive examination, during which he notes his "stethoscope is bobbing to the throbbing" of her heart, that he realises he is the cause of her racing pulse. At this point he becomes quite keen to reciprocate the affection.

The physician in popular song has almost always been male. But this is not so in Graham Parker and the Rumour's *Lady Doctor*, nor in Robert Palmer's *Bad Case of Loving You*: "Doctor, doctor, give me the news, I've got a bad case of lovin' you ... A pretty face don't make no pretty heart; I learned that ... from the start."

Avarice falls short of professional misconduct (and so is included in the 33% of songs we classified as "other") but is found in several lyrics. In *Like a Surgeon*, Weird Al Yankovic considers himself a failure and "the disgrace of the AMA" – but only because his "patients die before they can pay." In

The Doctor, Loudon Wainwright III is also cynical: "I went to the doctor and the doctor said ... Shucks ... you owe me 300 bucks. And you can call me in the morning, that is if you're not dead."

Doctors as carers or in need of care

A third of the songs reviewed portrayed the doctor in some form of caring or healing role, either literally in the case of bodily illness or, more often, metaphorically in the case of lovesickness or a broken heart.

Several songs portray doctors in their workaday role. John Mayall almost certainly had a sexually transmitted infection in mind when he wrote *Medicine Man*, while Harry Nilsson's *Coconut* is about curing a stomach ache. Health promotion, though, does not get an easy ride, as in Willie Nelson's *I Gotta Get Drunk*: "My doctor's telling me I gotta slow down. But there's more old drunks than old doctors. So let's have another round."

In *Alibi*, Slash is also inclined to ignore medical advice: "I feel alright, doin' what I do, I ain't gonna toe the line, not til I turn blue ... I ain't gonna waste a second, doin' what you say."

Bright Eyes' *Bowl of Oranges* is a rare example of the doctor being the one who needs help: "I came upon a doctor who appeared in quite poor health. I said 'There is nothing I can do for you that you can't do for yourself.' He said 'Oh yes you can, just hold my hand. I think that that would help.'" In the light of high suicide rates among the profession, increased understanding of this kind might be welcome.

Tunng's *Hands* also portrays potential vulnerability – a

doctor who has failed to save a patient stands despairingly in a corridor with his head in his hands.

Antipathy is more often portrayed than empathy. Richard Thompson's *Grey Walls* is a bitter critique of the incarceration and drug treatment of people with mental illness. The way psychoanalysis is portrayed is no more sympathetic, particularly its cost. The *Ballad of Sigmund Freud* by the Chad Mitchell Trio portrays a cynical view of how "a starving young physician trying to better his position" encouraged followers to see "there's gold in them there ills." In *Psychotherapy*, Melanie sings to the tune of the gospel hymn *When the Saints*: "Your analyst will cure you, long as you can pay the cheques … As the id goes marching on."

In summary, songs featuring doctors as suppliers of illicit drugs are less common than expected. If love is seen as an illness then we can expect doctors to be closely involved, especially given their expertise in matters of the heart. Emotional complexities arising from the intimacy of the doctor–patient relationship are reflected in songs portraying romantic attraction, and even the perception of sexual prowess.

Empathy for doctors is rare and they are at times presented as avaricious, although they are occasionally portrayed in caring and healing roles. But we can perhaps leave the last word to Bob Dylan, who clearly has respect for the profession. In *Motorpsycho Nightmare* the singer is accused of being a travelling salesman. "No," he says, "I'm a doctor, and it's true. I'm a clean cut kid, and I been to college too."

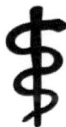

Back to the Future: How Good are Doctors at Gazing in the Crystal Ball?

British Medical Journal December 2006

The prediction in 1986 that a million people in the US would have AIDS by now was extraordinarily accurate, but the prediction that we would have a vaccine against HIV was wrong. The success of the predictions, or lack of it, may tell us the likely value of current attempts to foresee the speed and nature of medical advance: sometimes you have to look back to look forwards.

More than thirty years ago, in a study commissioned by the then Bristol-Myers company, 227 of the world's leading clinical scientists were asked to predict the state of medicine in the early 21st century. Among those interviewed were James Watson, who along with Crick discovered the double helix structure of DNA, Robert Jarvik, designer of the first artificial heart, Candace Pert, who helped identify endogenous opioid receptors in the brain, Michael DeBakey, a pioneering cardiac surgeon, and Michael Epstein, who identified the Epstein-Barr virus.

The scientists came from 10 countries (13 were from the United Kingdom), but most were based in the United States, so the US is usually the reality against which I test their predictions – but the conclusions should be widely applicable.

Curing cancer

Back in 1986, all the buzz in cancer therapeutics was about biological response modifiers. We were going to dissect out elements of the immune response, amplify them, and set them to work on tumours with devastating effect. Of course, it came to very little: interleukins, interferons, and even tumour necrosis factor proved sadly ineffective against common solid tumours and were unexpectedly toxic when given in pharmacological doses. In the mid-1980s there was great, if misplaced, faith in these agents. Despite this, future rates of cure were predicted accurately.

The pollsters told the specialists they interviewed that "the average cure rate for cancer patients of all types" was about 50%. They then asked what it would be in the year 2000. Estimates ranged from no change to 90%, with a median of 65%. Currently, the US Centers for Disease Control say that the overall five year survival rate for adults diagnosed with cancer in 1997–2002 is 65%.

Of course, surviving five years from diagnosis does not actually equal "cure": screening or improved diagnostics may simply start the survival clock earlier in the course of a disease that will ultimately be fatal. But calculating five year survival rates is standard practice in oncology, so the specialists in 1986 were probably using the "five year equals cure" convention when making their estimates.

Interviewees were also accurate in distinguishing between tumours for which survival would improve (haematological malignancies and breast, prostate and ovarian cancers) and those for which it would not (cancers of the lung, liver, stomach, and pancreas, and malignant brain tumours). The only big improvement they missed was in colorectal cancer.

Paradoxically, the specialists interviewed were wide of the mark when asked which treatments would be responsible for this improved outcome. Trastuzumab (Herceptin) and bevacizumab (Avastin) notwithstanding, neither in 2000 nor today [2006] is it monoclonal antibodies, "magic bullet" drug-antibody conjugates, or cytokines that are making the difference — nor is it anti-angiogenic and anti-metastatic agents, which the cancer scientists of 1986 had high hopes for. Improvements are due to earlier diagnosis, better surgery, better radiotherapy, better hormonal and cytotoxic chemotherapy (including use in the adjuvant setting), and better supportive care.

The potential of cancer vaccines was also overestimated: 60% of those polled thought that by 2000 we would be vaccinating people "directly" against certain types of tumour — but we still have no effective vaccine treatment for established cancers. And, with the exception of a vaccine to prevent cervical cancer (approved in autumn 2006) and immunisation against hepatitis, we still have no vaccines against oncogenic viruses.

In short, oncologists in 1986 were remarkably accurate in predicting improvements in overall and tumour-specific survival, but for entirely the wrong reasons.

Matters of the heart

The clinical scientists were also prescient in cardiology, even when it came to identifying the precise means by which progress would be effected — unlike the oncologists. Perhaps precision as to means is easier when the problem is basically faulty plumbing rather than myriad derangements in the processes controlling cell division and differentiation.

How good are doctors at gazing in the crystal ball?

Cardiovascular experts in 1986 identified a bright future for thrombolytics: almost half rated their promise as 9 or 10 on a 10 point scale. This was bold.

The interviews took place six months after publication of the 12,000-patient GISSI trial, which showed that patients with myocardial infarction treated with streptokinase had an 18% reduction in mortality at 21 days. But this was two years before publication of the ISIS-2 study, which many regarded as the required confirmatory trial. In 1986, streptokinase was the only clotbuster available. Given the possibility of uncontrolled bleeding, many clinicians worried about the balance of risk and benefit; and even in 1988 there was still no consensus that thrombolysis should be routine.

Those interviewed in 1986 were right about the limited potential of implanting an artificial heart: 90% said that transplants would be preferred for the foreseeable future. They were also correct in spotting balloon angioplasty as a technique with plenty of room for expansion. In 1993, angioplasties overtook coronary artery bypass grafting among Medicare patients, and now twice as many angioplasties (1.2 million) as coronary artery bypass grafts are performed annually in the US. But panel members were not correct in thinking that the number of bypass grafts would show a corresponding sharp decline. Numbers rose steadily from 230,000 in 1986 until peaking in 1997. Although bypass grafts have declined 10% since then, half a million are still carried out each year.

For coronary disease prevention, it's surprising that a third of those interviewed did not expect doctors in 2000 to be advising their patients to limit consumption of cholesterol. On the other hand, more than half rated research into lipid metabolism and transport as 7 or higher on the scale of future promise, a year before the first statin was licensed by the Food and Drug Administration.

Rather optimistically, 69% thought that general nutritional advice would have improved the problem of obesity by 2000. Asked about the likely health status of the population, the panel did not foresee burgeoning rates of overweight and associated problems such as diabetes and cardiovascular disease.

HIV and other infections

Biotechnology, cancer, and infection specialists were asked in 1986 how many people in the US would have developed AIDS by 2000. The median estimate was 1.1 million. The latest cumulative total (for 2004) is 944 000. Given the many uncertainties of the time, the 1986 estimate was extraordinarily accurate. But the success of an HIV vaccine was overpredicted: 60% thought we'd have a safe and effective vaccine by now.

It's difficult to judge whether the scientists were right about antiretroviral drugs: interviewees were asked to say when an "effective cure" would be "generally available." Does chronic suppression of viral load count as success? Did "general" availability include the developing world? Just over half (52%) thought we'd have a generally available and effective cure by 2010.

Perhaps because of the eradication of smallpox in 1977, vaccines were accepted as the best way forward in combating infectious disease in general. Hepatitis was judged most likely to see significant advance, but not herpes or malaria. Right in all respects. The panel also did well in their forecast for measles: only 17% said there was a reasonable chance of eliminating the disease by 2000. Measles worldwide still causes half a million deaths each year.

Nervous system

More than 80% of the neuroscientists interviewed thought that stimulating nerve cell growth and regeneration would be clinically viable by 2000 and that we would be using genetic engineering to treat inherited disorders. Seventy per cent predicted that fetal brain tissue transplants would be an accepted treatment and would be "very effective" for at least a few neurological conditions.

A lot closer to the mark were their expectations about how more traditional treatments might develop. The hope that a new generation of atypical antipsychotics would carry a much reduced risk of causing movement problems (extrapyramidal side effects and tardive dyskinesias) seems to have been realised. Those interviewed were right in thinking that traditional psychoanalysis would be a relatively unimportant element in the treatment of mental illness, but that use of cognitive therapy would increase. No one predicted a comeback for electroconvulsive therapy.

They were also right in thinking that any progress against Alzheimer's disease would, at best, be modest. Only 10% thought we would be close to curing Parkinson's disease. And we are not.

Artificial bits and bobs

Though the scientists were right in predicting that the next 15–20 years would see a greatly expanded role for artificial

Correct and incorrect predictions

Oncology
Right
- Two thirds of patients cured (alive five years after diagnosis)
- Progress piecemeal
- Best improvement in survival in breast cancer and with leukaemias and lymphomas
- No real change in cancers of lung, liver, pancreas, stomach, central nervous system

Wrong
- Progress will come through antibodies, cytokines, vaccines
- No real change in survival in colorectal cancer

Cardiovascular disease
Right
- Thrombolysis becomes routine
- Angioplasty takes off
- Lipid metabolism research highly promising
- Little potential for implantable heart
- Little promise in minimising neuronal damage after stroke

Wrong
- Decline in coronary artery bypass grafts
- Nutritional advice improves problem of obesity

Infectious diseases
Right
- Cumulative total of close to 1 million AIDS cases in US
- Vaccines against hepatitis but not against herpes and malaria
- No cure for common cold

Wrong
- Safe and effective HIV vaccine by 2000
- Cure generally available by 2010 (assuming chronic suppression of viral load does not count as cure)

Nervous system
Right
- Little progress against Alzheimer's disease and Parkinson's disease
- Cognitive therapy used more
- Reduction in tardive dyskinesia

Wrong
- Fetal tissue transplants, and gene repair, accepted and effective
- Less dependence on opiates for severe pain

knees and hips, they were wrong in thinking that the same would be true for artificial wrists, ankles, toes and fingers and artificial skin and blood. (In the mid-1980s, there had been a brief but well-publicised spurt of research into the idea that blood could be replaced by oxygen-carrying fluorocarbon emulsions. But the idea never came to much clinically.) The panel also had misplaced faith in the imminent importance of implantable drug infusion systems, and in a bright future for penile implants. No one in 1986 saw Viagra coming.

Lessons for the future of futurology?

It didn't take medical degrees a mile long to predict that the major health problems in the West would be those associated with ageing, or that malnutrition and infections would continue to plague the rest of the planet. Other questions must have required very careful consideration, and some, such as the cumulative number of AIDS cases in the US and the overall cure rate for cancer, were answered with surprising accuracy.

Treatments that did not achieve the success predicted
- Immune modulators in cancer
- Drugs to regenerate neurons
- Fetal tissue transplants
- Genetic engineering for inherited disorders
- Artificial blood
- Implanted drug infusion systems

Where predictions erred, they did so by being overoptimistic. In predicting that vaccines would quickly be successful against HIV, clinical scientists were extrapolating from a history of solid achievement against other pathogens. But in predicting the widespread use by 2000 of cytokines, therapeutic antibodies, genetic engineering for inherited disorders, fetal tissue transplants and artificial blood, they were being carried away by the enthusiasms of the moment.

Whether this "flavour of the month effect" tells us something specific about medical scientists or something general about being human is an open question. But the demand for predictions will not dry up. Overall, what this set of crystal ball gazers got right is more surprising than what they got wrong.

Index

3TC 33

Abortion 150, 198–202
ACE inhibitors 57–61
Acetylcholine 173, 205
Ackerman, Michael 10, 12
Acyclovir 39
Adams, Gerry 71, 72
Addiction 165, 173
Addenbrooke's Hospital 8, 27, 54, 140
Adjuvant therapy 147
AIDS 30–36, 78, 153, 212, 216, 218
Akerstedt and Gillberg 142
Albert, Jan 34
Alcohol 168, 189–92, 206
Alzheimer's Disease 60, 148, 217
Amanita muscaria 203–6
Ambridge 144–54
Analgesia 201–2
Angina 178
Angiogenesis 125
Angioplasty 45, 47, 117, 215, 218
Antenatal screening 183
Antibodies 126, 134
Antipsychotics 217
Aorta, aortic aneurysm 80–82
Archers, The 144–54
Arthritis, juvenile 147
Ashford Hospital, London 185, 187
Atheroma 48–50

Auden, WH 167
Auto-eroticism 165–6
Avastin (bevacizumab) 214
Ayemenre, Clara 185
AZT (zidovudine) 31, 33, 34, 36

Baird, Maclean 82
Baker, Robin 101–3
Balkwill, Frances 133
Banks, Ian 76, 78, 79
Barnes, Charles 15
Barton, Simon 39
Bashford, Lindy 75
BBC 144, 152, 153
Beard, Richard
Beatles, The 207, 208
Beck, Aaron 99
Beddington, Rosa 196
Bergler Edmund 166
Beta blockers 58
Biological response modifiers 131
Bipolar disorder 83–8
Birkbeck College 168
Birmingham University 27, 113, 116
Birth, birth rates 147, 199
Blake, William 108
Blankenhorn, David 50
Bone marrow banks 121–23
Boreham, Mr Justice 63
Bowel cancer 136
Bradford University School of Pharmacy 60

221

Brahms, Diana 20
Brave New World 193
Breast cancer 126, 132, 138, 147, 156
Brenner, Barry 59
Bristol-Myers 212
Bristol Royal Infirmary 117
British Cardiac Society 43
British Heart Foundation 55, 82
British Medical Association (BMA) 26, 64, 139, 140
Broadbent, Donald 142
Brown, Louise 194
Brunel University 14
Burkitt, Denis 155–6
Burt, Sir Cyril 107

CCNU (lomustine) 62–9
Caerphilly 158–9
California Supreme Court 20
Cambridge University 15, 16, 22, 103
Cancer 145–7, 213–214
Cardiac deaths 145–6
Cardiomyoplasty 114
Cell lines 13–21
Chamberlain, Douglas 55
Chattur, Dr 139
Chemotherapy 125, 135
Chelsea and Westminster Hospital 39
Chernobyl 121–23
Chickenpox 37, 41
Cholesterol 49, 50, 215
Chronotherapy 135–38
Cigars 163, 164
Cigarettes 160–75
Circadian rhythms 135

Circumcision 201
Civil partnership 151
Claridge, Gordon 85–7
Clark, David 94–5
Clark, Leland 116
Cloning 20, 193, 194
Clotbusters 43
CML 126
Cocaine 165, 185–6, 189
Cognitive Behaviour Therapy (CBT) 93–5, 98–100, 217
Cohen, Leonard 297, 208
Coley, William 130
Collison, Pamela 62, 63, 67, 69
Colon cancer 155
Consent 22–29
Constipation 155–6
Cooke, Kieran 8
Corey, Larry 38, 39
Coronary artery disease 42–50, 178
Coronary artery bypass (CABG) 50, 178, 179, 215, 218
Cortex, cortical development 200–02
Cortisol 199
Costall, Brenda 60
Covid-19 30, 32
Creativity 83–8
Crisis in Men's Health 78
Croom, David 67
Customs and Excise 185–9
Cyclosporin A 53
Cytotoxics 125–6

de Bono, David 44, 46
Defibrillators 54–7, 148

Index

Delamothe, Tony 80
Depression 97–100, 152, 165
Derbyshire, Stuart 199
Dermatology 181
Desmond, Julian 34
Diabetes 57–60
Diet 48, 155–6, 157, 216
Diogenes syndrome 89–93
Doctor-patient communication 182–4
Dolly the sheep 194
Dorman, Richard 71–2, 74
Douglas, John 14–15
Down's syndrome 152, 154
Drug smuggling 185–9
Drumm, Brendan 158
Dudley Road Hospital 26
Dylan, Bob 211

Elizabeth Garrett Anderson Hospital 25
English, Terence 54
Ether 192
European Collection of Cell Lines 18
European Union 143
Extrasensory perception 103–9
Eysenck, Hans 109–112

Faithfull, Simon 117
Father Christmas 203–6
Fell, Dame Honor 16
Fentanyl 201
Fibre 155–6
Fibrillation 55
Fisk, Nicholas 198, 199, 201
Fluorocarbons 115–17, 219
Fly agaric 203–6

Foetus, foetal pain, surgery 193–7, 198–202
Folie à deux 66
Fowler, Godfrey 169
Fowles, John 88
Franks, David 16
Freud, Sigmund; Freudian 100, 164–8, 170, 211
Frontal lobe 90, 91, 92

Gaddum's Pharmacology 190
Gale, Robert 122–23
Ganzfeld 104–5
Gastric cancer 156
Gay men 78
Genentech 129, 131
General Medical Council (GMC) 23, 25, 64
Genes, gene mutation 33, 83, 86
Genetic engineering 128–29, 218
Gerard, Brendan 195, 197
Gey, George Otto 14, 17
Glasgow Western Infirmary 157
Glivec (imatinib) 126–7
Golde, David 19
Gorbachev, Mikhail 123
GPs 70–80, 151–4, 148, 180–4
Gosden, Roger 195, 196, 197
Guardian, The 207
Gynecology teaching associates 25

Hammersmith Hospital 182, 194
Harefield Hospital 54
Hartviksen, Gjermund 181
Health economics 176–9

Heart attack 42–7, 55, 145, 146, 182
Heart failure 112
Heart transplant 54, 176, 178, 207
Heart-lung transplant 51–4
Heather, Brian 82
Heathrow Airport 185–9
HeLa cells 13–21
Helicobacter pylori 156–9
Hendron, Joe 72–4
Heparin 48
Hepper, Peter 201
Herceptin (trastuzumab) 126
Heroin 185, 186
Herpes 37–41, 216
High blood pressure 58–60
Highly Active Antiretroviral Therapy (HAART) 31
Hip replacement 153, 176, 178
HIV 30–36, 78, 153, 212, 216, 218, 220
Holland 43, 44
Howe and Summerfield 168
Hrushesky, Bill 137–8
Human Tissue Act 2004 21
Huxley, Aldous 193

Iceland 83
ICI 132
Illegitimacy 151
Illingworth, Roger 49
Imatinib 126
Immortalisation 18, 19
Immune system 129–31, 138
Immunomodulators 128, 219
Immunosuppression 53

Imperial Cancer Research Fund 133, 158
Inhalation 173, 190–2
Institut Pasteur 34
Institute of Psychiatry 170, 174
Intelligence, IQ 109–111
Interferon 18, 129, 131, 133–4
Interleukins 130, 133
In vitro fertilization 193

Jack Daniels whiskey 190
James, William 89
Jerrigan, Joseph Paul 12
Jochelson, Waldemar 205
Johns Hopkins University 14, 16
Johnston, Peggy 35
Jones, Ernest 164
Jones, Howard W 14
Joyce, James 86
Junior doctors 139–43

Karlson, JL 84
Keady 71
Kennedy, Ian 23–4
Kidney disease 57–60, 178
King's College, London 23, 112
Kipling, Rudyard 135
Kirschvini, Joseph 103
Kretschmar, Robert 24
Kuwabara, Yoshinori 194–5, 197

Lack, Henrietta 13–16
Lancaster University 203
Langston, Bill 119–20
Leeds University 195
Levi, Francis 135–7
Lippman, Marc 138

Index

Lomustine (CCNU) 62–9
Loren, Sophia 207, 209
Lovastatin 49
Luesley, David 27, 29
Lundbeck 68
Lymphocytes 35
Lymphokines 19, 130
Lymphotoxin 129–31

Manchester University 101
Marré, Michel 59
Marsden, David 120
Marshall, Barry 159
Matarazzo and Saslow 168
McColl, Kenneth 157
Medical Ethics Today (BMA) 26
Medical Research Council (MRC) 21,
 MRC Applied Psychology Unit 106, 141, 142
Microalbuminuria 59, 60
Middlesex Hospital 38
Monoclonal antibodies 134
Montaner, Julio 30
Montgomery 154, 181
Moore, John 19, 20
Mortality rates 144–6
MPTP 118–21
Muscarine 205
Mushrooms 203–6

National Heart Hospital, London 47
National Institute for Allergy and Infectious Diseases 35
National Institutes of Health 40

NHS 124, 176, 177, 179
NICE 179
Nicotine, gum, patches 160–75
Northern Ireland 56, 70–4, 192
Nowers, Mike 90, 91
Nucleoside reverse transcriptase inhibitors 31

Oliver, Michael 43
Opiates 173, 199, 218
Oral eroticism; personality 166–8, 170, 173
Ovarian cancer 137
Oxford University 48, 85, 169, 183

Panic attack 93–5
Papworth Hospital 51–4
Parkinson's Disease 118–21, 217
Parving, Hans-Henrik 58, 59
Patel, Raj 38–40
Pendleton, David 183
Philpot, Michael 91, 93
Pitts Crick, Jonathan 117
Pit viper, American 57
Plath, Sylvia 83, 85, 87
Porter, Cole 209
Professional patient 23, 24
Prostitutes 34
Prozac 92
Pryor, Ruth 85
Psychiatry 181
Psychoanalysis 166–8, 211
Psychokinesis 106, 107
Psychosis 84–8
Pulmonary hypertension 52

Quality-Adjusted Life Year 176–9
Queen Charlotte's Hospital 198, 200, 201
Queen's University, Belfast 201

Radiology 181–2
Radiation 122–23
Rape 151
Reindeer 204–5
Reitano, Mike 40
Reitz, Bruce 51
Rickards, Anthony 47, 48
RJ Reynolds 171
Robinson, Jean 25, 28
Rolling Stones, The 207
Rotterdam 44
Royal College of General Practitioners 183
Royal Society of Medicine 30
Royal South Hampshire Hospital 38
Russell, Michael 170, 171

Salmons, Stanley 112–114
Salt, Patrick 116
Sandoz 19
Santa Claus 203–6
Sargent, Carl 103–9
Sauna 191
Schizophrenia 64–6, 83–8
Seattle 56
Seligman, Martin 96–8
Sellers, Peter 207
Sepsis 149
Serotonin reuptake inhibitors 92
Shaman 203–6

Shearer, Raymond 73–4
Sherr, Lorraine 183
Shumway, Norman 51
Siberia 203–4
Sikora, Karol 129, 133–4
Skloot, Rebecca 21
Sleep loss 139–43
Smoking 160–75
smoking machines 160, 161
Smith, Steve 27
Smyth, Chris 149
Snuff 172
Society for the Protection of the Unborn Child 195, 197
Souhami, Robert 66
South Armagh 70
Sowton, Edgar 57
Spier, Ray 18, 19
Spitzer, Victor 10–12
Statins 48–50, 216
St Mary's Hospital 27
St Nicholas 204
Stem cell harvest 122
Stents, coronary 46–8
Straus, Stephen 40
Streptokinase 44–5, 215
Suicide 76, 77, 145, 146
Surawy, Andrew 79, 80
Surawy Stepney, Nick 207
Surrey University 18
Surrogate patients 25
Swedish Institute of Infectious Diseases 34
Swyer, Gerald 25

Taberner 191
Tamoxifen 132

Index

Tar 161, 170, 171, 172, 174
Targeted drugs 125–28, 131
Taylor, Rogan 203, 206
Telemedicine 180–2
Thomas, Dylan 85, 88
Thrombolysis, thrombolytics 43–5, 215, 218
Tizzard, Juliet 196
Tobacco 160–75
Trastuzumab (Herceptin) 126, 214
Tromso 181
Tufts University 156
Tumour Necrosis Factor 128–31, 133–4

Ulcers, stomach; duodenal 156–9
University of Bristol 191
University of California 19
University of Colorado 10
University of Pennsylvania 114
University of Southern California 50
University of Washington 38
University of Warwick 183
Urine drinking 205

Vaccines 36, 40, 41, 214, 216, 218
Vaginal examination 22–9, 187
Vaping 7, 160, 162, 175
Varicella 37
Vegetarians 156
Viagra 219
Vickers, Paul 62–9
Vickers, Margaret 62–9

Victoria Station 55
Videophone 180
Viruses 13, 30–41
Visible Human Project 9–12

Wakeford, Richard 8, 22
Waldegrave, William 153
Wain-Hobson, Simon 34
Wallwork, John 42, 53, 54
Ward, Patrick 70–71
Warneford Hospital, Oxford 94
Warren, Robin 159
Wasson, RG 205
Watkins, Gwen; Vernon; Tristan 84
Watson, James 212
Weaning 167–8
Well Man clinic 75
Well Woman clinic 75
Wellcome Foundation 18
Whitburn, Vanessa 152, 153
Whitlock, David 10
Wilkinson, Bob 141
Williams, Alan 178–9
Williamson, Peter 77, 78
Winston, Robert 194
Womb, artificial 193–7
Women's Health Concern 25
Woolf, Virginia 87
Wynn-Jones, John 148, 152–4, 180–2

York University 178
Yorkshire Ripper 63, 68

Zidovudine (AZT) 31, 33, 34, 36
Zucker and van Horn 167

Books by Rob Stepney

Smoking: Psychology and Pharmacology (with Heather Ashton), Tavistock, 1982; *Cancer: What it is and How it's Treated* (with Howard Smedley and Karol Sikora), Basil Blackwell, 1985; *Heart disease: What it is and How it's Treated* (with John Wallwork), Basil Blackwell 1987; *Good Pubs of Oxford* (with Dave Perry), Pintsize Press, 1990, 1992 and 1995; *Good Pubs of Cambridge* (with Dave Perry), Pintsize Press; 1991; *A Funny Way with Words* (with John Lanyon, Adrian Lancini and Edward Fenton), Wychwood Press, 2012; *Words go out to Play* (with Adrian Lancini, Edward Fenton and John Lanyon), Charlbury Press, 2018; *Does Nothing Rhyme with Charlbury? Poems from a Little Town of Stone* (editor), Wychwood Press, 2006; *Because We Never Said Goodbye* (editor), Wychwood Press, 2008; *Spirit of People and Place* (editor), Walcot Books, 2020.

In 2002, in what was described by Margaret Drabble as "a heroic act of publishing", Walcot Books republished a revised edition of *Owen Glendower* by John Cowper Powys. This edition was subsequently bought by Overlook Press, Woodstock, New York.

About the author

Rob Stepney has an MA in psychology and philosophy from Oxford University, an MSc in pharmacology from the University of Newcastle-upon-Tyne, and a PhD from the Cambridge University Department of Medicine.